Beyond the Clinic Walls

Beyond the Clinic Walls

CASE STUDIES
IN COMMUNITY-BASED DISTRIBUTION

James A. Wolff
Robert Cushman, Jr.
Florida A. Kweekeh
C. Elizabeth McGrory
Susanna C. Binzen

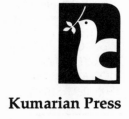

Kumarian Press

Book Design and Typesetting   Alan G. Yost

Acknowledgments   The authors would like to thank the following people for their cooperation, support, and contribution to the development of these case studies:

Cecelia Nemah	Aloysius Taylor	Gabriel Hina
Peter Hne	Nettie Prall	Edith Scott
William Gibson	Marion Roberts	Dorothy Dakaboi
Edwin Zahn	Doris Walker	Cecelia Taplah
Julia Sherman	William Johnson	Muftau O. Falade

This book could not have been written without the insight, guidance and tremendous energy of Wokie Stewart, who provided the authors with invaluable assistance. Deirdre Strachan and Marilyn Edmunds of the Pathfinder Fund also provided extraordinary support during the preparation and for the publication of these cases. The authors would also like to thank Leslie Curtin and John Howard of the United States Agency for International Development for their encouragement and efforts on behalf of this book.

Special thanks go to Linda Suttenfield for all the attention and advice she has provided the authors during every stage of this book's development.

This work was funded by the United States Agency for International Development under contract number DPE-3039-C-00-5075-00.

Copyright © 1990 Kumarian Press, Inc.
630 Oakwood Avenue, Suite 119, West Hartford, Connecticut 06110-1529 USA

Printed in the United States of America

94   93   92   91   90   5   4   3   2   1

Cover design by Margaret Heagney

Library of Congress Cataloging-in-Publication Data

Beyond the clinic walls.

    "Published in association with Management Sciences for Health."
    Includes bibliographical references (p.   ).
    1. Birth control--Africa, West--Case studies. 2. Birth control clinics--Africa, West--Case studies. 3. Community health services--Africa, West--Case studies. I. Wolff, A. James, 1947-
HQ766.5.A358B49   1990   363.9'6'0966   90-5281
ISBN 0-931816-08-4

Table of Contents

Introduction   vii

Part I   **(A)**   **Community-Based Distribution -- Overview**   1

       (B)   **Republic of Momonboro -- Background Data**   6

Part II   **Planning**   10

     Case 1   Reaching Out to Underserved Populations:
The Decision   14

     Case 2   Mobilizing Resources for the Project:
Getting Support   24

     Case 3   Research and Planning for the Project:
Leaving Nothing to Chance   31

Part III   **Information for Effective Management**   37

     Case 4   Developing an Information System:
Dealing with Data   41

     Case 5   Setting Targets and Giving Feedback:
The Jeffersonville Supervisory Meeting   54

     Case 6   Collecting and Using Data:
Mr. Krumah's Dilemma   60

Part IV   **Supervision**   66

     Case 7   Conducting Effective Group Supervision:
The Royalton Supervisory Meeting   69

Part V   **Compensation and Pricing**   77

     Case 8   Developing Financial Incentives:
The Sales Force   79

Part VI   **Financial Control**   86

     Case 9   Designing a Financial Management System:
Keeping an Eye on the Money   89

Part VII   **The Community-Based Distribution Start-Up Kit**   106

     Complete Checklist   137

Annexes

1 Chronology of Events: The Community-Based Distribution Process 140

2 Sample Job Descriptions 142

3 Sample Forms 149

4 Training Program for Community-Based Distribution Agents 153

5 Flipchart for Family Planning Presentation 156

6 Community-Based Distribution Agents' Oral Contraceptive Checklist 158

Bibliography 160

Index 162

INTRODUCTION

This book contains a series of case studies which depict the management issues a family planning organization faces in designing and implementing a new community-based distribution (CBD) program for contraceptives. The cases, which take place in the fictional country Momonboro, are based on an actual program initiated in an African country, and reflect the problems and successes which that program experienced. The authors chose to record the experiences of an African CBD program, first, because there is growing interest for community-based distribution of family planning services in many African countries, and second, because the authors wished to explore the particular characteristics and challenges of designing and implementing a CBD program in that region.

The cases in *Beyond the Clinic Walls* were developed for managers who are either contemplating or engaged in the process of designing and implementing a CBD program. For these managers the book can serve as:

- a guide to program development, exploring in some detail crucial issues in the design and implementation of CBD program management;

- a training resource, providing case studies and analyses of the case studies for use in workshops and small group discussions on CBD program management.

Beyond the Clinic Walls is divided into seven sections.

Part I(A), COMMUNITY-BASED DISTRIBUTION -- OVER-
VIEW, discusses the factors which are necessary to manage a successful community-based distribution program. Part I(B), REPUBLIC OF
MOMONBORO -- BACKGROUND DATA, provides demographic
and economic information on Momonboro, and a description of the
organizations which are central to the family planning program.

Part II, PLANNING, explores the important areas of strategic
planning, operational planning, and assessment of the internal and
external environments in a family planning organization and the
country. This section also includes a primer on CBD program
management.

Part III, INFORMATION FOR EFFECTIVE MANAGEMENT,
addresses the issues and challenges of establishing an effective CBD
management information system. The areas covered in this chapter
include the design of effective information flows, the type of data to
collect for CBD programs, and the analysis and use of management
data at different levels in the program.

Part IV, SUPERVISION, examines how effective supervision can
improve staff performance.

Part V, COMPENSATION AND PRICING, challenges the common
notion that family planning services should be provided free. This
section explores the issue of charging for contraceptives and examines
the factors to consider when pricing contraceptive products in a CBD
program.

Part VI, FINANCIAL CONTROL, demonstrates how an effective
but not overly burdensome financial control system is developed and
then revised to best meet the program's needs and work within the
program's constraints.

Part VII contains a CBD Start-Up Kit, which will serve as a guide
through the major tasks of planning and implementing a CBD project.

The annexes contain sample job descriptions for every position in the
CBD program, sample forms used for data collection, the curriculum
of a training program for CBD agents, the checklist used by CBD
agents to determine a client's suitability for oral contraceptives, and
the contents of the flipchart used by CBD agents when they make
their family planning presentation to potential acceptors. There is also
a chronology of the events surrounding the CBD program in the
fictional country of Momonboro.

Each of the sections of the book begins with an overview of the basic concepts demonstrated in each case. Following the overview, the cases are presented in a narrative form. Written to depict realistic management situations or problems, they illustrate the application of the management concepts addressed in the section. Each case is preceded by a series of learning points to guide the reader to the major issues addressed in the case. These learning points will be particularly useful for managers who wish to adapt this material for training workshops. Each case is followed by a Case Analysis that discusses the problems presented in the case. In two of the chapters, the cases have been divided into more than one part.

Beyond the Clinic Walls may be used in a number of ways:

- **Trainers** may use sections of the book to develop modules for training in key CBD areas. The background material and case learning points can be tailored to the workshop format and provide guidelines for development of training objectives or group discussion points. The cases accompanied by the case analysis will provide material for trainers and allow training participants both to share their own family planning experience, and to build on the information and experience depicted in the case.

- **Managers** interested in the development of a CBD program in Africa may wish to read the cases sequentially and then study them in more detail in the case analysis section. In this manner, they may find it easier to compare the specific areas covered in the design and implementation of CBD programs with the situation in their own country. On the other hand, they may wish to read the book straight through following the history of the design and implementation of an African CBD program.

- Other readers may wish to use the book as a **reference** in critical areas of CBD management, identifying common problems in CBD management and exploring possible solutions to them.

The cases in this book are based on real situations. As such they record actual management problems faced by real managers. It is impossible to describe in this kind of book all the skills necessary for effective CBD program management. The authors hope that readers will complement the information and experience recorded in these cases with their own family planning and managerial experience. A creative integrative process drawing on the reader's skills and experience, as well as the case materials, will increase the usefulness of this book.

PART I (A)   COMMUNITY-BASED DISTRIBUTION

Overview

This handbook is about planning and implementing a community-based distribution system. Community-based distribution (CBD) programs reach beyond the clinic walls to provide contraceptives in the communities where people live. The ultimate goal of all CBD programs is to improve the accessibility of contraceptive services and supplies. There are four primary ways in which a CBD program does this:

Geographic   by bringing the source of services and contraceptives closer to where people are;

Economic   by ensuring that contraceptives are affordable;

Administrative   by making it as convenient as possible to obtain and use contraceptives;

Cognitive   by providing information that is accurate, reliable and understandable so clients can make informed choices about the method they wish to use.

The following section explores some issues which are particularly relevant to planning and implementing a community-based distribution program.

Official Support

It is important to get input and support from appropriate authorities and ministries. In many situations, there is resistance from the medical community to non-medical personnel prescribing and distributing contraceptives. The approval of medical personnel is critical to overcoming such procedural obstacles, and also to establishing linkages for support and referral. This is a vital component of any CBD program. Involving and getting support from local physicians and other health personnel can also help to legitimize the program within the community.

Community Support

A critical factor in starting a community-based distribution system is involving the community in the planning process. A needs assessment should be conducted to determine: current usage; awareness of and demand for contraceptives; community perceptions; and the level of interest in such a program. As with any community development program, it is vitally important to involve local leaders, including health and family planning workers, from an early stage. This will provide valuable information on how best to design and implement the system, and will also involve the community in the process so they will support the program.

Selection of Distributors

Community perception of a CBD program and its legitimacy can often be dependent on the person who is selected as the distributor. This is, therefore, a crucial factor in the success of the program. The distributor should be known and respected in the community. Community leaders and other groups can help to suggest potential candidates. Specific characteristics to look for in distributors will vary depending on the situation. However, in many programs it has been found that older women who are married, are mothers, and are themselves satisfied contraceptive users are effective distributors. Often it is personality traits such as confidence, sensitivity, and enthusiasm which are the most important characteristics.

Training

The training which distributors receive will also vary considerably by program and by the kind of work they are expected to do. In most programs, training sessions will be relatively short but intense. At a minimum, distributors should receive training and practice in basic physiology, how the specific contraceptive methods which they will be distributing work, and effective ways to approach and communicate with people in the community. They should also be given information about how the whole CBD program will work, including the resupply and record-keeping systems. A very important part of training is the correct use of checklists to assess the safety of a method for each individual client, and to know when to refer a client to a professional health provider in case of complications or for clinical methods.

Supervision

Supervision is a critical part of any health program. Because they have limited training and are often isolated, it is particularly important to monitor and support community-based distributors through effective supervision. Supervision should be supportive and instructive rather than critical. Ideally, supervisors should visit distributors where they work. However, because of logistical and transportation problems, this is not always possible. Holding meetings for distributors at which their performance is discussed and monitored can also be effective. (Supervision will be discussed in more detail in Section IV).

Remuneration

Many different systems have been tried to compensate community-based distributors for their work. These have involved both monetary and non-monetary compensation. In some programs, distributors have been given a small salary. However, this is difficult to sustain in many areas due to limited budgets, and can also create problems in motivating workers to carry out their tasks. The most common system is to allow distributors to keep a certain percentage of the revenue they earn from sales of contraceptives. In other areas, non-monetary recognition and minor rewards have enabled programs to operate successfully with volunteers.

Resupply Systems

Resupply systems will vary greatly depending on the specific geographic and logistic factors which exist in a particular program area. Availability and reliability of transportation, distance from the distribution point, and availability of proper storage will greatly affect the system which is devised. The existence of a reliable and operational resupply system is one of the most critical factors to a successful CBD program, particularly in remote rural areas. This system will be closely linked with the system of record-keeping and supervision which are devised for the program.

Pricing Contraceptives

Pricing of contraceptives is a controversial aspect of CBD programs. In many countries, contraceptives are subsidized by the government or international donor agencies. As sustainability of programs has been given increasing attention, pricing for cost recovery has been explored as a strategy. In many programs where distributors are paid based on a percentage of sales, the price of contraceptives will be an important factor in devising a remuneration scheme. Pricing has clear implications for affordability and accessibility of services to the poorest sectors of society. The acceptability of charging for contraceptives, and the implications for program sustainability, accessibility, and worker compensation need to be carefully considered in formulating a pricing strategy.

Mix of Services

In some community-based distribution programs, family planning services and supplies are offered as part of more comprehensive health care or development assistance programs. In some cases, this has increased the acceptability and motivation of people to use family planning. These positive benefits need to be carefully weighed and considered in the context of specific programs, and evaluated against the ability of the program and the distributor to effectively provide a range of services.

Contraceptive Method Mix

In many countries, the mix of contraceptive methods which CBD workers can provide will be determined largely by policies set by the Ministry of Health or other government organizations. While there has been some resistance to the provision of services by nonprofessionals, evidence increasingly shows that if distributors are properly trained and supervised, there is little risk associated with the provision of non-clinical methods by nonprofessionals. In most CBD programs, pills, condoms, and foam are methods which can be purchased or obtained from the distributor. She or he is also trained to refer potential clients to a health facility for clinical methods such as the IUD or surgical procedures.

Socio-cultural Implications for Community-Based Distribution Programs

Many women in Africa have hectic fifteen-hour work days in which they have to do housework, farming, marketing, and care for their families. It is very difficult for a woman who is this busy to travel several miles to a clinic for family planning. If she makes the first visit, she might not be able to find the time for the second visit. In addition, men tend to be the major decision-makers in the area of family planning, so that after a woman has struggled to find the time to come to the clinic and be counseled on various contraceptive methods, she may say, "I want the method, but I have to tell my husband." A CBD program addresses both of these problems: the CBD agent comes to or works near the woman's home, so she does not have to travel, and the CBD agent can counsel both husband and wife together. Moreover, CBD programs provide modern contraceptive methods which are ideal substitutes for the traditional family planning method of abstinence, which is becoming less popular as societies modernize and become more urban.

Family Planning CBD Experience

Community-based distribution programs have been used in many countries and contexts for a number of years. While there are clearly some limitations to such systems, there is evidence that, given appropriate and careful planning and supervision, such programs can effectively provide services and supplies to communities which otherwise would not have access to family planning services. There is an increasing body of literature on the experience and lessons learned from such programs. You will find a bibliography with references in the back of this book.

PART I (B)   THE REPUBLIC OF MOMONBORO
Background Data

Geography and Demographics

The fictional Republic of Momonboro is located on the west coast of Africa, and has a land area of about 43,000 square miles. Its thirteen counties and three territorial areas have a population density of about thirty-five persons per square mile. Six of the thirteen counties border the coast. The seven inland counties have a large geographic area, where most of the agricultural production takes place.

By most standards, Momonboro ranks as one of the poorest countries in the world. The average monthly income is about sixty momambi (approximately sixty U.S. dollars). Its population, estimated at about two and a half million people, struggles between the pull of the few urban centers and the need to make a living in its rural, agriculturally based economy. In the capital city of Placatte, there is a growing population of urban poor.

The population of Momonboro is comprised of sixteen distinct tribal groups; of these, three dominate national political and economic activity. Approximately 10-15 percent of Momonboro's people are Christian, 15 percent are Muslim, and the remainder follow traditional religions.

Health and Family Planning Statistics

As in many developing countries, it is difficult to find reliable data on health. In the absence of hard data, the following estimates of basic health indicators have been made.

Child Mortality rate	45/1000
Maternal Mortality rate	4.9/1000
Infant Mortality rate	144/1000

A recent national nutrition survey showed that in rural areas nearly a quarter of all children under five years of age exhibited signs of chronic undernutrition.

Other serious threats to health include cholera, malaria, measles, tuberculosis, and gastroenteritis, which are the five leading causes of hospitalization in Momonboro. Malaria is the most common outpatient disease, leading the second most common, parasites, by a 4 to 1 margin. The leading causes of registered deaths in each of the last four years were pneumonia, malnutrition, anemia, and gastroenteritis.

The economic and social pressures of unregulated fertility continue to be a serious problem in Momonboro. The total fertility rate has been estimated at 6.7 children per woman. Contraceptive prevalence is roughly 8 percent. The national rate of population growth is estimated at 3.3 percent.

The Ministry of Health

The Ministry of Health (MOH) is responsible for the delivery of health care services at a national level. All hospitals, both private and public, are certified by the MOH, which also runs the national drug service and appoints medical directors to government hospitals. In recent years, financial difficulties have caused the ministry to reduce many of its services. It has been increasingly unable to provide any services to many parts of the country, and has encouraged the private sector and private voluntary organizations to provide hospital and other health services.

Because family planning is a health service, it operates under the authority of the MOH. The MOH has authorized the Family Planning Association of Momonboro (FPAM) to help it broaden its family planning service base. The MOH pays rent and utilities for the FPAM headquarters, and ensures that FPAM has duty-free privileges. The MOH also runs maternal and child health/family planning (MCH/FP) clinics that FPAM supplies with essential drugs and contraceptives. Staff in these backup clinics are paid by and work under the MOH. These clinics serve as a referral network for the limited number of FPAM field workers. FPAM is responsible for training the MOH MCH/FP staff in family planning.

Attempts to address its health and population problems are seriously compromised by Momonboro's deepening financial crisis. The MOH has seen a steady erosion in its budget over the last five years. Drugs and other commodities are in extremely short supply.

The Family Planning Association of Momonboro (FPAM)

FPAM has been in existence for more than twenty years with a volunteer-based structure. The Member's Assembly, its highest organizational body, meets every two years to elect officers, review the association's activities and attend to administrative matters. The National Executive Committee is elected at this meeting and reports to the members. Serving under this body are committees for finance and administration, and programs. These committees meet once each quarter and make recommendations to the Executive Committee. FPAM also has paid senior staff who sit on the Executive Committee as ex officio members.

The organization has branches in nine counties. At each branch there is a Local Executive Committee, as well as finance and administration and program committees. These groups monitor the activities of paid field staff who in turn report directly to national level coordinators for Information, Education and Communication (IEC) Programs.

FPAM operates a family planning clinic in the capital city of Placatte. It also has a small-scale outreach program conducted by two community field workers. They serve as motivators, conduct educational activities, and refer patients to the clinic for care and contraceptives.

Through its clinic in Placatte, FPAM provides a variety of services, including client counseling and supplying contraceptives. It also performs laboratory work to screen for contraindications for certain methods, as well as testing for reproductive tract infections. In addition, it provides clinical contraceptive services, including IUD insertions. Referral for voluntary sterilization procedures are made to the nearest hospital.

FPAM also has many programs currently operating in Information, Education and Communication. These include programs in family life education in schools for students and teachers, production of regular radio programs in local dialects using national networks, and development of audiovisual family planning materials. The IEC unit also conducts regular IEC sessions at MCH/FP clinics, and supports a mobile unit for community motivation.

FPAM is involved in a number of special projects, including peer group counseling through the National Youth Program, a women in development project in cooperation with Planned Parenthood, and programs for young teenage girls through 4-H Clubs.

The organization also has a number of training programs. It provides training for all family planning service delivery providers from the Ministry of Health. FPAM also supports the training activities of other national and international organizations in Momonboro.

FPAM receives 85 percent of its operating budget from International Assistance for Child Spacing. The remainder is raised locally through volunteer fund-raising drives, inputs in kind from the MOH, and recently through the sales of contraceptives. Outside of its regular operating budget, FPAM solicits funds for special projects. Pathways and Global Family Planning Assistance are currently funding special projects.

Pathways

Pathways is an international family planning organization based in Washington, D.C. in the United States, with a regional office for Africa in Nairobi, Kenya. Pathways has assisted FPAM for many years by providing technical assistance as well as funding for training and special projects.

PART II   PLANNING

Overview

Planning is central to many of a manager's tasks. It is needed to ensure that the organization appropriately defines both its broad role and a specific way to accomplish its work. Planning is necessary for many purposes within an organization. It happens in different ways and at different levels. This section will outline several different types of planning, some issues which managers need to keep in mind to plan effectively, and the role they should play throughout the planning process. This discussion will help you to evaluate the events and decisions in Cases 1 through 3.

Basic steps in the planning process include:

- Assessing the situation
- Selecting important issues
- Analyzing the environment
- Setting goals, objectives, and targets
- Identifying and addressing opportunities and obstacles

Planning activities can be divided into two broad categories: strategic and operational. We will discuss both types, starting with strategic planning.

Strategic Planning

Strategic planning is concerned primarily with the long-term goals and strategies of the organization. Good strategic planning should answer the following questions:

WHERE is the organization now?

WHERE do we want to be in five to ten years?

WHAT are we trying to achieve?

HOW can we get there?

Strategic planning is concerned with defining the two most general parts of an organization's plan:

> The *Mission* of the organization, which is the broadest, most complete statement about the central purpose of the organization;

> The *Goals,* which are general statements which reflect the factors which are required to achieve the organization's mission. A goal describes what you expect to accomplish by a particular point in time.

In many larger organizations, strategic planning takes place at a very senior level. However, in smaller organizations, such as many which deliver family planning services, it may involve staff members. In organizations of any size, it is important for the staff at all levels to know and support the organization's mission and goals.

Operational Planning

Operational planning translates the broad ideas formulated in the strategic planning process into more specific terms which can be put into practice. It outlines in practical terms how the resources of the organization will be utilized to achieve its mission. To do this, a plan must define:

> *Strategies,* which describe HOW each goal will be achieved. To determine the most efficient and effective strategy, it is useful to explore several alternatives. The staff should be involved in generating ideas and helping to select which strategy will work best.

> *Objectives,* which are statements that describe the specific results to be achieved, when, and by whom for each strategy, so that a goal can be met. This is the first step to making the ideas raised as missions and goals operational. To be useful an objective must be:

>> Specific -- so that its meaning is clear to everyone

>> Attainable -- so that staff will be motivated to strive for it

>> Measurable -- so that activities can be evaluated

> *Targets,* which help you to measure the performance of your staff and your program in meeting your objectives. Targets must be expressed in specific, numerical terms.

The Environment

All parts of the planning process require information about the environment in which the organization operates. These can refer to both *external* factors, which are outside the organization, and *internal* factors, which are within the organization.

Some examples of each include:

Internal	*External*
staffing	economy
budget	political climate
structure	demographic factors

For a family planning program, some specific examples of relevant environmental factors are:

External
- societal views of contraception
- groups which may influence the success or failure of program, such as:
    religious and community leaders
    women's organizations
    traditional birth attendants and other health workers
    formal medical sector
- health and family planning data
- government goals and policies regarding population
- physical environment/constraints

Internal
- level of integration or separation from other health programs
- infrastructure available and necessary
- existing programs in health and family planning

Sources of information about these issues are varied. They can range from official census statistics to more informal information from discussions with local groups, community leaders and members of the community which the program will serve. Often this kind of less formal information can be extremely useful, as it outlines important and relevant issues that formal reports may miss. Knowing about and addressing these issues can be vital to the success of a program.

After listing and examining the relevant environmental factors, the manager needs to determine which are obstacles and which are opportunities for his or her program. Opportunities are important resources, either material or otherwise, which should be used to benefit the program.

Obstacles are more complicated to deal with. They can include shortages of resources such as personnel or supplies, geographic and infrastructure barriers, and social or religious values which will stand in the way of your program. Obstacles can be systematized into groups: those which can be solved, those which can be reduced, and those which you must work around.

Another important use of information will be to help you anticipate and plan for problems which may emerge in the future. By being aware of these potential problems, you can devise ways to either avoid them, address them early before they become problems, or be prepared for them when they arise.

At all stages in the process of planning and implementing a program, it is important to seek input from the people who will influence its success. This includes people in appropriate ministries or funding agencies; those who work with similar programs; the staff of your own program or organization; and members of the community which the program is designed to serve.

Soliciting and using input from this broad range of people serves two important functions. First, it allows you to utilize an important resource: the suggestions and perspectives of people from all levels of the process. Second, when the program is implemented, this interaction will foster cooperation among people who must work to ensure its success. If they have been involved in the planning process, they are much more likely to support both the goals and structure of the program.

The following three cases present the experiences of a private family planning organization as it devises a plan to more effectively fulfill its mission. At the end of each case, you will be asked to answer several questions to evaluate how the situation has been or might be handled. You should use the information you have just read about planning to help you.

Note: Before using these cases, be sure to carefully read the previous section "Background Data -- The Republic of Momonboro."

CASE 1:   THE DECISION

Case Learning Points

- Understand how to use demographic and programmatic data to identify important problems and prepare a strategic plan.

- Be able to identify a number of different strategies for delivering family planning services.

- Determine what information is needed to assess the feasibility of different strategies in particular contexts.

A) Case Study: The Decision

Mrs. Kokie Tyler sat sandwiched between Sam Ford and James Alexander in the back of a rented minibus. All passengers on the bus were en route to the opening reception of the annual meeting of the West African Family Planning Association, and they were in good spirits. Today also marked Mrs. Tyler's first anniversary as Executive Director of the Family Planning Association of Momonboro (FPAM). In the back of the bus, with the wind from the open window in her face, she thought about the past year.

An accountant by training, Mrs. Tyler had started working with FPAM as a volunteer twelve years ago. When she became Executive Director, the organization was in the bleakest period of its nineteen-year history. It had been red-lined by its funding agency for poor performance and its continued existence was uncertain. Shortly before Mrs. Tyler was asked to become the Executive Director, an independent evaluation had forced a reexamination of the organization's practices, financial management system, and service delivery capability. As a result of this evaluation the former director, along with a number of senior management personnel, had resigned.

"Not the best situation in which to start a new job," Mrs. Tyler thought wryly. But things had worked out well. Within three months she had appointed a new director of finance, implemented an efficient financial management system, recruited new staff, and started to build a cohesive and collegial senior management team. She had worked particularly hard at building and strengthening relationships with the Ministries of Health, Planning, Education, and Information and felt that this was beginning to pay off. Though these efforts had been successful and the organization's clinic was operating at capacity, she was still dissatisfied with the impact FPAM was having on its real mission: delivering family planning services to women of reproductive age.

Her thoughts were momentarily interrupted as the minibus pulled into a petrol station to refuel. Taking advantage of the lowered noise level, Sam Ford jokingly asked her if her "charisma had won over the women of Momonboro." "Not yet," she replied, "but we're working on it." Before she could go on, the minibus started up again and the drone of the engine made it impossible to continue the conversation.

Several months earlier, Mrs. Tyler remembered, she had begun to visit communities within the capital city of Placatte and in the surrounding rural areas. She had taken long walks through the shanty towns of the city and its environs, talking to family planning field workers and people she encountered in the street. She was surprised to find that the level of knowledge about family planning was high. In fact, most mothers knew about modern methods of contraception and indicated that they understood the importance of child spacing. These observations were confirmed by a demographic study that had been conducted by an international organization and the Ministry of Planning and Economic Affairs (see tables 1-5).

In the following weeks, Mrs. Tyler had visited a sample of women who had been referred to the clinics by the field workers. She found that although they all had expressed interest in using modern contraception, very few had actually visited the clinic. When questioned as to why they had not followed up by going to the clinic, the women cited the long wait, the high cost of transportation, loss of time from domestic responsibilities, and long distances between home and the clinic.

When they arrived at the hotel, Mrs. Tyler took the opportunity to renew her conversation with Sam. Sam was a staff member of Pathways, an American family planning organization which had worked with FPAM since it was founded. "How long have we known each other, Sam?" Mrs. Tyler asked.

"Must be ten years," Sam said.

"You've been helping us out at FPAM for even longer than that, and I need some help on a new initiative that I've been thinking about. I've been looking over our statistics, and they're not impressive. We're generating a great deal of interest in modern methods, but we're not getting the clients to the clinics. We need to develop a better way of reaching clients, and we need your help."

As they walked through the hotel lobby, Mrs. Tyler continued, "I'll put together some of the information that I've been collecting. If you could look at them sometime tomorrow, we could discuss it over dinner tomorrow night."

"Kokie," Sam said smiling, "You'll use every chance you get to make me work."

Study Questions

1. Using the information from the case and the tables, what kinds of programs might best help FPAM to fulfill its mission?

2. What strategies might Kokie Tyler and Sam Ford develop?

3. For each strategy that you have suggested, list the key points that you would have to consider to assess its feasibility in Momonboro.

Table 1

Reproductive Intentions of Women in Union

Age	Total	Want No More Children	Want to Space*	Want Next Child Soon*	Want Child, Undecided When	Does Not Know	Number of Women Surveyed
Total	100.0	17.1	33.4	31.2	10.6	7.5	3536
15-19	10.4	1.5	39.3	36.4	13.5	9.3	366
20-24	19.3	6.8	43.3	34.9	8.3	6.7	684
25-29	24.0	9.1	42.5	31.2	10.9	6.3	849
30-34	15.1	19.3	32.6	27.3	11.6	9.2	535
35-39	14.9	25.6	23.4	27.8	12.3	11.0	526
40-44	7.5	34.3	12.4	34.4	10.4	8.6	264
45-49	8.8	47.3	11.6	23.2	13.0	4.9	312

* "Wants to space" means wants next child two years or more from now; "wants next child soon" means wants next child within next twenty-four months.

Table 2

Knowledge of Family Planning Methods, Where to Obtain Them and Current Use

Method	Percent Who Know Method		Percent Who Know Source*		Percent Who Ever Used		Percent Currently Using	
	AW	IUW	AW	IUW	AW	IUW	AW	IUW
Any Method	74	71	48	44	21	17	8.9	6.5
Any Modern Method	72	69	45	43	16	15	7.0	5.6
Pill	64	61	43	38	16	13	4.9	3.4
IUD	32	31	24	20	3	3	0.9	0.7
Injection	44	42	30	28	3	2	0.3	0.3
Vaginal Methods	10	8	10	8	1	1	0.2	0.2
Condom	30	26	21	16	4	3	0.2	0.1
Female Sterilization	43	45	29	28	1	1	1.0	1.1
Male Sterilization	6	6	4	4	0	0	0.0	0.0
Any Traditional Method	33	28	11	10	9	8	1.4	1.1
Periodic Abstinence	18	12	11	9	4	3	0.9	0.6
Withdrawal	16	15	--	--	4	3	0.2	0.1
Traditional Methods	13	14	--	--	1	1	0.3	0.2

AW -- All Women (Number Surveyed = 5214).

IUW -- In-Union Women (Number Surveyed = 3536).

*   For periodic abstinence, this refers to a source of information for the method.

Table 3

Reasons for Non-use of Family Planning *

Reason for Non-use	Percentage
Number of Women Surveyed	1523
Fear of side effects	12
Opposed to family planning	4
Partner objects	5
Religion	3
Too costly	6
Difficult to obtain	8
Not sexually active	4
Doesn't know methods	12
Breastfeeding	33
Menopause/subfecund	4
Other	11

* Among non-pregnant non-users who report that they would be upset if they became pregnant soon.

Table 4

Current Users of Modern Family Planning Methods by Source and Type of Method

Source	All Modern Methods	Supply Methods*	Clinical Methods*
Number of Users	347	261	86
Total	100.0%	100.0%	100.0%
Government Hospital or Clinic	28.8%	21.0%	56.1%
Church Hospital or Clinic	6.6	2.9	17.1
FPAM Clinic	43.7	48.3	12.4
Private Doctor or Clinic	5.2	4.3	8.1
Pharmacy/Shop	13.0	20.3	0.0
Field worker	0.5	0.6	0.0
Other	1.8	2.1	1.5
Doesn't know	0.4	0.5	0.0

* Supply methods include pill, injections, vaginal methods, and condoms. Clinical methods include the IUD and female and male sterilization.

Table 5

Percentages of Women Who Are Currently Using Any Method and Any Modern Method of Family Planning

Characteristic	Any Method	Any Modern Method*	Number of Women Surveyed
Total	8.4%	7.0%	5214
Age			
Less than 30	8.4	7.0	3227
30 and Over	8.4	6.9	1987
Number of Living Children			
0-2	6.8	6.2	3184
3-4	10.9	7.7	1166
5+	11.1	9.3	863
Urban-Rural Residence			
Urban	13.7	11.1	2044
Rural	5.0	4.3	3170
Region			
Greater Placatte	8.4	6.6	109
The Hedeg	4.0	3.9	269
Rest of Country	8.2	7.3	4835
Educational Status			
No schooling	3.1	2.6	3311
Some primary	5.3	5.1	931
Primary completed	25.1	20.4	971
Reproductive Intentions**			
Wants no more	17.0	14.2	605
Wants to space	7.6	6.6	1181
Wants next soon	1.3	1.3	1103

*   Modern methods: Pill, IUD, injection, vaginal methods, condom, female and male sterilization.

**   Restricted to women currently in union.

B) Case Analysis: The Decision

Identifying Problems

Several important observations can be made based on the survey data contained in Tables 1-5:

1. Basic knowledge about family planning is high: 70 percent of all Momonborian women have heard of at least one modern method, particularly the pill.

2. A significant percentage of women (17 percent) say they do not want to have any more children, and one-third would like to postpone their next child for at least two years.

3. Despite these high levels of contraceptive awareness and interest in child spacing, less than half the women know where they can get a family planning method. Less than 20 percent have ever used contraceptives, and only 9 percent are currently using any method. Interestingly, 40 percent of the unprotected women said they would be upset if they were told in the next few weeks that they were pregnant.

4. When asked why they did not use family planning, these women cited a variety of reasons (see Table 3). A significant proportion of these could be addressed through a more focused community program. For example, greater and more complete information could assist the 24 percent who either don't know of any methods, or fear side effects. Making contraceptives more geographically and financially accessible could eliminate the obstacles for those who cite that they are difficult to obtain (8 percent) or too costly (6 percent).

What the survey data shows is a substantial gap between potential demand for contraceptives and the provision of appropriate services. Based both on the information in the tables and on Mrs. Tyler's informal surveys, a significant reason for non-use seems to be that services are not accessible.

Only a small percentage of the population, 9 percent according to the survey, currently uses contraceptives. A look at service distribution (Table 4) shows that the majority of these services are provided at two centers in Placatte, the FPAM clinic and the Government Hospital clinic, and that the provision of services in other locations or sectors is negligible.

From the background material, it is also clear that the areas outside the capital, where 75 percent of the people live, are largely underserved. The fact that only 14 percent of urban women report current use of contraceptives raises the question of how accessible the two large clinics are to the urban population.

As Mrs. Tyler sees it, the problem is clearly one of underservice in the face of potentially high demand. Furthermore, she knows from her own discussions and interviews with clients and women in the communities that accessibility is a big problem in the city, and may be one of the primary obstacles to providing effective family planning services.

Identifying and Exploring Potential Solutions

How might family planning services be expanded in Momonboro? Some possibilities include:

1. Expanding the services provided at existing clinics.

2. Adding satellite clinics to the existing infrastructure, either as separate family planning clinics or integrated into existing ministry or private health services.

3. Exploring and implementing new types of programs, such as community-based distribution, social marketing or commercial sales programs.

Assessing the Alternatives

FPAM could try to increase the capacity of the two large clinics. However, from the case and the background material, we know that they are already working at capacity. More importantly, Mrs. Tyler knows from the statistics and her interviews that for many potential clients, these sites are not readily accessible. Therefore, this alternative will not help to address the most important issues -- informing people about family planning and getting services out into the community where the clients are.

One possible solution is to develop a number of satellite clinics in communities throughout the city. This could possibly be done through the existing Ministry of Health infrastructure. While this would help to overcome the problem of inaccessibility, it is not clear that there are sufficient resources to establish and staff such clinics. FPAM clinical staff are working at capacity in the existing clinic, and cooperative efforts with the Ministry are concentrated on training and routine maternal and child health services. Because of the fees they charge, any efforts made with private physicians would exclude a major target group -- the urban poor. This alternative also does nothing to provide more and better information about family planning methods.

What is needed here is a novel approach to a difficult problem, an approach which improves education and access, is community-based, and relies relatively little on existing resources which are already being used to capacity.

One kind of program which should be explored is a community-based distribution (CBD) program. Community-based distribution programs have been increasingly used to provide family planning and other health services to communities in which, for a variety of reasons, clinic-based services are not feasible or are not adequate. Some factors which may indicate that a community-based distribution system should be explored are: geographic isolation; poor coverage of a community by traditional, clinic-based health services; shortages of trained personnel and other resources; cultural barriers to contraceptive use; and demonstrated demand for services which is not being met.

Mrs. Tyler feels that with foreign funding and technical assistance she can start a CBD program which will quickly become self sufficient. The feasibility of this idea should be explored. Important questions to be considered include:

- Can FPAM get cooperation from the community and the support of key community leaders and other important individuals for such a program?

- Will they be able to recruit, train, and motivate CBD workers?

- Can FPAM supervise the program and also provide the necessary clinical support?

Some specific considerations for establishing a community-based distribution system will be discussed in the following section.

CASE 2:   GETTING SUPPORT

Case Learning Points

- Practice gathering and using information necessary to undertake a needs assessment of a community.

- Understand the importance of planning and public relations for community development projects.

A) Case Study: Getting Support

Kokie Tyler's dinner presentation was short but comprehensive. Sam Ford agreed with her interpretation of the data. Mrs Tyler's analysis indicated that inaccessibility of services and lack of information were the major obstacles facing FPAM in delivering family planning services to Momonborian families. After discussing several alternative strategies, Mr. Ford and Mrs. Tyler agreed that an outreach and community-based distribution program would help FPAM to reach these families. Mr. Ford returned to Washington convinced of FPAM's commitment to establishing such a program.

Over the next six months, conversations and negotiations between FPAM, donors and the Ministry of Health took place. A foreign-funded maternal and child health/family planning (MCH/FP) training project was winding down. Several other foreign-funded population initiatives, especially in the area of policy development, were experiencing some success. This therefore proved to be a good time for a reevaluation of Momonboro's population strategy, and two years ago a team of consultants came to Momonboro. Their mandate was to review the country's experiences in population and family planning. On the basis of these findings, they were to provide recommendations for a Plan of Action to serve as a guide for future population program activities.

Mrs. Tyler had always maintained an open door policy, and she made a great effort to assist the assessment team. Her cooperation and input enabled her to help to shape the report. The team's findings also confirmed her thoughts that an outreach program held the greatest potential for improving the provision of family planning services.

The assessment team came to the unanimous conclusion that the demand existed for greatly expanded services. They determined that the existing infrastructure was adequate to build on, and that government and private sector interest in expanding service delivery was strong. Post-partum programs in maternity centers and clinics, community-based distribution of contraceptives, and sale of contraceptive products through the commercial sector were identified as important possible vehicles for service delivery.

The report also confirmed many of the observations Mrs. Tyler had made during her discussion with Mr. Ford.

"While there appears to be considerable demand for family planning services, especially in Placatte, the number of acceptors resulting from the efforts of the community outreach workers is unimpressive. For example, only sixty-five new acceptors last year were attributable to the efforts of field workers. This was in large part the result of there being only two field workers to cover an urban population of 250,000 people.

"There is also some confusion over the extent to which field workers can become on-going suppliers of contraceptives. While they provide the initial disbursement of pills, it is unclear if they have been given a mandate to resupply continuing users."

The report went on to recommend:

"Field workers should be trained and motivated to work with local leadership structures to set up a network of community-based distribution points. An information system needs to be worked out so that all clients who have been motivated by field workers to accept family planning are credited to the program. Providing field workers with payment based in part on the number of acceptors could be a useful incentive for dramatically increasing results."

Shortly after the recommendations of the assessment team had been reviewed, Mrs. Tyler wrote to a number of international family planning funding agencies about her idea. Among these letters was one addressed to the Africa regional representative for Pathways.

"We have decided to expand our family planning program with your support and assistance. Specifically, we are looking to establish community-based distribution services in the greater Placatte area and its immediate surroundings. In light of this, we are writing to request your immediate reaction to our proposal. We appreciate Pathways' willingness to assist FPAM on a larger scale. We have worked very successfully with Pathways on smaller projects in the past, and look forward to a close working relationship in the future.

"You might be interested to know that the initial grant which enabled FPAM to begin operations in 1956 was the amount of 100 momambi given through Mrs. Edith Drinkwater of Pathways."

This letter to Pathways brought the swiftest result; one month later Mrs. Tyler received a reply to her letter from Professor Pedipaw, Pathways' Regional Representative, stating that he had submitted her preliminary request, together with his comments, to the central office in Washington for review. He also assured her that he would do his best to visit Momonboro as soon as possible to review the situation, discuss the alternatives, and begin the process of developing a proposal.

Professor Pedipaw came to Momonboro that September, and met with the senior staff of FPAM. Together they reviewed the situation and drafted guidelines for the development of a proposal. He also requested that FPAM conduct a needs assessment in the planned project service area to serve as a basis for drafting the final proposal.

Study Questions

1. What information would you like to obtain for your needs assessment of the target communities? Where would you get this information? Outline types of information you would need, and prepare some sample survey questions which could be used.

2. What can you do to improve the chances for approval of your CBD program at Pathways? In your own organization, FPAM? In the community?

B) Case Analysis: Getting Support

Needs Assessment

The needs assessment has four main objectives:

1. To identify the community's family planning needs;

2. To assess and understand the community, including its demographic structure, existing services, and administrative and political structure;

3. To determine whether a particular community should be selected for a project and, if so, how the program should be introduced to maximize its chances of success;

4. To directly involve the community and its leaders in the program from the planning stages.

Needs assessments can be conducted in a number of ways. Community surveys can help to provide information on perceptions and attitudes within the community. However, they are difficult to design and costly to administer.

Often there are some data already available. In this case Mrs. Tyler has already determined that an unmet demand exists by using the national demographic survey and FPAM service data, along with her own informal on-site interviews.

If one determines that a small local survey is warranted, existing questionnaires can often be used directly or with minor modifications. In this case, Mrs. Tyler could use the national survey questionnaire to find out specific information for some select districts of Placatte being considered as potential sites for the CBD program.

A further step in the needs assessment is to determine what family planning and health care services already exist in a particular area. This is important as there is no need to duplicate existing services. Furthermore, it is important to identify other key players, both to coordinate service provision and to encourage cooperation. Often services can be combined or made to complement each other in cooperative efforts. For example, starting a CBD program will most likely mean that some people will be referred for medical exams, resulting in a greater case load for the local government clinic. Enlisting their cooperation and involvement early in the program planning stages is important. Alternatively, there may be obstacles which need to be identified well in advance.

The needs assessment should also focus on the target population and local demographics. Useful information will include: total population; number of households; ethnic and religious makeup; existing transportation services; and basic geographic and administrative information.

These data are important for planning both the kind of program which would be appropriate, and how it might best be implemented. The program manager might decide to select one area over another for a pilot project because it is more manageable, thus giving the program a greater chance of success. Alternatively, one might select CBD agents on the basis of ethnic or religious affiliation for particular neighborhoods. Agent zones should follow natural geographic or demographic boundaries.

Planning and Public Relations

Mrs. Tyler has demonstrated her planning and public relations skills in a number of areas. In the first case, we saw that she established and maintained contact with a number of important ministries and agencies. In this case, she has demonstrated an active role in contacting and involving foreign donors. She has adopted an aggressive attitude towards Pathways. Although such an approach is risky, it allows her to set the tone of their discussions.

Mrs. Tyler also got very involved with the in-country evaluation, and has influenced the consultants' perceptions of the family planning situation in Momonboro. The outcome and recommendations of the evaluation are therefore likely to assist her efforts to gain support for a CBD project. This was an important step in preparing for the project proposal and in getting support for it.

Mrs. Tyler now has to apply the same skills to her own organization and the community at large.

Mobilizing one's own organization to support a new project can often be very difficult. While the project may promise something new and effective for a community, people within the organization responsible for implementation may perceive it differently. There is generally resistance to change in any organization, and for a staff that is already working to capacity, there is always a fear of being overwhelmed with new responsibilities.

Mrs. Tyler also has to mobilize the communities in which the project will be implemented. Of particular importance is gaining the support and involvement of the community leaders who can then have a multiplier effect on the broader public. While FPAM already has a good working relationship with them, both national and local level ministry and political leaders need to be encouraged to support the new project. Specific strategies for getting support from these sectors will be explored in the next case. Special attention should be paid to officials of the Ministry of Health as they must sanction and accredit the program.

CASE 3:   LEAVING NOTHING TO CHANCE

Case Learning Points

- Understand the relationship between effective planning, management style, and program effectiveness.
- Identify specific strategies for getting support for a program.

A) Case Study: Leaving Nothing to Chance

Mrs. Kokie Tyler leaned back in her swivel chair, the air conditioner humming loudly in the background. Professor Pedipaw's visit had been a great success, and Pathways seemed to be clearly committed to supporting the new outreach project which Mrs. Tyler had proposed. Things had moved much more quickly than she had anticipated when she had initiated this important new phase in FPAM's programs. It had taken less than one year to achieve what she had optimistically predicted would take two. However, despite her current satisfaction she knew that there was no time for complacency. "Now for the hard part," she thought to herself. Scribbling on a yellow pad she began to sketch out the things which she needed to accomplish in the next three months.

Internal

- Motivate and involve FPAM staff
- Set up a planning committee
- Assign tasks
- Develop a survey for needs assessment and baseline planning data
- Get a formal proposal ready

External

- Select and mobilize specific communities
- Get support of Ministry of Health
- Get support from other sectors
- Establish close working relationship with USAID
- Ensure visibility through good media coverage
- Investigate opposition to nonmedical distribution of pills

Making initial contact and developing relationships with communities was a formidable challenge. First, Mrs. Tyler had to identify communities to survey, and then develop a survey instrument. Her staff agreed that the technique of using the survey to initiate contact and build relationships with the communities offered major advantages.

In the next several weeks, Mrs. Tyler and her staff selected six potential low-income target communities using the national housing service survey. Three were in greater Placatte, and three in outlying areas. They then prepared a baseline survey to identify population, households, ethnic groups, religions, size of the area, zones, sub-divisions, public transport, administrative structures, and existing health and family planning service facilities. The survey questionnaire was sent to and later picked up from the mayor in each community. The survey also asked the leaders for ideas regarding selection criteria for agents, as well as suggestions about how they might be deployed.

When the survey was completed, FPAM held a meeting at its head-quarters for the mayors and commissioners of each community to discuss the results. At this meeting Mrs. Tyler and her staff also outlined the plan to establish community-based distribution of contraceptives in these communities. They asked the commissioners for suggestions, and enlisted their help.

At the same time, FPAM was seeking support from the Ministry of Health (MOH) for the program. FPAM already had ties to the Ministry though its clinical family planning service delivery, supplies, training and Information, Education and Communication efforts. For the previous six years, FPAM had been a key actor in the development of national curricula for health workers and paramedics for maternal and child health/family planning (MCH/FP) training.

Several meetings were held with officials from the MOH. These discussions covered a wide range of issues, and eliminated some of the barriers to implementing an urban CBD program. For example, there was considerable concern about the distribution of contraceptives by people who did not have formal medical training. Fortunately, a new primary health care program which had been introduced two years before was changing attitudes about pharmaceutical dispensing because it permitted distribution of ten basic drugs by nonmedical personnel. Although several MOH staff thought that nonmedical distribution of oral contraceptives was unethical and dangerous, serious opposition to the program did not develop. A compromise was reached whereby community agents would use a checklist to screen clients for contra-indications before distributing the first cycle of pills.

In January of the previous year, Mrs. Tyler and her staff had been ready to develop the final draft of the proposal. Two Pathways consultants were due to visit Momonboro to assist them. Mrs. Tyler decided to use the consultants' visit to generate public support for the project. She arranged national television coverage of their arrival at the airport, and called an "emergency meeting" of FPAM's senior staff on Sunday night to welcome the consultants and to map out their scope of work. Over the next few days the consultants visited the Ministry of Health and several other ministries which were connected with the project. They were well-received during their visits with community leaders. This contact permitted them to get a realistic perspective of the community's needs to incorporate into the proposal, as well as generating support for the project among the many sectors involved.

Study Questions

1. Using the information from the last three cases, outline the factors you see as effective or ineffective in Mrs. Tyler's planning of the CBD program.

2. Do you think Mrs. Tyler is an effective manager? Why?

B) Case Analysis: Leaving Nothing to Chance

This case describes Mrs. Tyler's handling of a situation in which she needs to enlist the support of numerous different actors to successfully implement a complex new program. Together with the previous cases, it illustrates the planning process of the CBD program.

Mrs. Tyler clearly understands the complexity and the multiple levels of the planning process. She has gone to great lengths to ensure that it goes smoothly.

As a result of her previous assessments of the situation, Mrs. Tyler knows about the needs and the existing services, and is comfortable that the new program she has proposed is appropriate. In this case, she is interested in determining which communities should be targeted, how to plan the program implementation, and how to get the endorsement and cooperation of leaders at different levels.

She first used existing information (the national housing service survey) to identify the low income communities in Placatte and the surrounding areas as possible target areas. To study the potential sites and involve local leaders, she informed the mayors about the development of the project proposal. They were asked to complete the survey giving basic information about their jurisdictions. Their sense of involvement was also fostered by asking them to suggest criteria by which to select the community based distributors.

Mrs. Tyler used the survey skillfully not only to collect information about the communities, but also as a means of getting the cooperation of the local politicians. She provided feedback on their suggestions by scheduling follow-up meetings to discuss the project and the survey results with the mayors and other community leaders. Finally, she orchestrated the consultants' visit so that it became a major public relations event.

While she was working with the prospective communities, Mrs. Tyler was also seeking support from the MOH. Not only did she wish to involve the MOH and get its endorsement, but in effect she had to win approval for the distribution of contraceptives by non-medical personnel. This was achieved through a combination of her diplomatic and managerial skills, and the good fortune of the recent innovations in primary health care programs. It is interesting to note that there was reluctance within the MOH to approve contraceptive distribution, and a compromise was reached which involved the use of a checklist for contraindications plus a medical referral.

Mrs. Tyler also involved her own staff effectively. They worked with the visiting consultants to plan the project. Many of the staff were involved in conceptualizing the program, and therefore shared in the evolution of the proposal and the project. Mrs. Tyler therefore made it clear that the project was to receive high priority within FPAM.

This case outlines the importance of identifying potential problems early, and coming up with innovative and appropriate methods of involving people and institutions in the process. This not only provides important feedback and information, but also solicits the involvement and cooperation of numerous players. Their approval and cooperation will be crucial to the eventual success of the program. This case also illustrates the importance of being prepared and willing to negotiate and compromise, and to develop creative alternative solutions.

In summary, these cases demonstrate Mrs. Tyler's appreciation for and skills in planning and management. She understands the importance of detailed planning, setting goals and deadlines, involving all parties early on, and identifying potential pitfalls in advance. She also understands and uses public relations. She is a strong leader and exhibits a great deal of enthusiasm. This pervades the organization, with positive implications for the potential success of the project.

PART III   INFORMATION FOR EFFECTIVE _____ MANAGEMENT

Overview

The next three cases address the issues and challenges of establishing a good management information system for FPAM's community-based distribution program. A management information system (MIS) provides data and feedback to permit organizations to operate effectively. This system is essential for monitoring, evaluating and regulating the performance of individual staff members as well as the impact of the program as a whole. Each of these functions will be discussed below.

The MIS also provides information for inventory and resupply. In many programs, the MIS generates information for external use. This can include data such as contraceptive prevalence rates for a central statistical unit, and information on program performance for reporting to funding agencies.

One of the primary challenges of a management information system is ensuring that all necessary and relevant information is collected and utilized at minimal cost. Financial, technologic and staff costs need to be considered.

Conceptualizing and designing an MIS can be a long and detailed process. The system should be carefully thought through and discussed with all the people who will use it. This should include people who will gather the data, as well as those who will use the information for decision making. To the extent possible, the MIS should incorporate the various interrelated functions of the organization such as financial control, evaluation, resupply, staff monitoring and supervision, and reporting. It is very important that the MIS be flexible enough to allow for modifications as the needs of the program or users evolve.

One of the most important things to keep in mind when designing an MIS is to streamline the information which is gathered. It should be kept as brief and concise as possible. To determine what appropriate and important information the MIS should provide, the users of the system at each level should be identified. It is useful to begin by looking at what decisions are actually made in the organization, who makes these decisions, and what information they need in order to make good, intelligent decisions. This process will help to determine what information is necessary at each level of the organization, as well as what should be sent along to the next level of administration.

It is particularly important in a decentralized system such as a CBD network for the information to be used at the level where it is collected. This has several important implications. First, it can permit an individual agent to monitor his or her own performance. Secondly, it can be useful to compare the performances of people with the same responsibilities. Finally, when the information's usefulness is demonstrated, it reinforces the importance of collecting data which is timely and accurate.

Evaluation

Program evaluation is a central component of program management. Relevant and reliable information is essential for evaluating a program. Unfortunately evaluation in many programs is often only done by outside consultants at the middle or end of funding cycles. No one would question the importance of an external evaluator or of the need for funding agencies to evaluate the projects they sponsor. However, this process tends to reduce management's commitment to evaluation and to remove it from the day-to-day operation of the program.

Ironically, internal evaluation efforts are often susceptible to similar problems. Typically, management delegates the responsibility to one individual or a team, who are then perceived as a threat as they play a policing role, but they have no direct involvement or stake in the day-to-day activities. This method of evaluation runs the risk of becoming counterproductive.

For evaluation to be effective, management must build commitment to its importance and foster a sense of ownership in the process. The ideal first step is to lead by example, and for management to get actively involved in the promotion and conduct of evaluations.

When evaluation is integrated into the structure of a program, it usually occurs continuously and at many levels. In a CBD program, this may include self-evaluation by distributors, evaluation of agent performance by supervisors, and an internal or external evaluation team assessing the program as a whole. It is important for the specific

criteria by which the program will be evaluated to be clearly
determined at each level, and that the necessary information be
available.

Indicators

The selection of particular measures, such as indicators of individual
or program performance, has important implications. Some indicators
used in family planning and CBD programs are:

- numbers of client contacts

- new users

- active users

- dropouts

- clinic referrals

- average length of client contraceptive use

- quantity of sales of different methods

These measures are often made into ratios, such as new users per
client contact, so that the effectiveness, as well as quantity, of a
particular activity can be assessed.

Often targets are set for these indicators. Targets can be useful to
motivate individuals, as well as to direct programs. They can also
provide a standard against which performance can be evaluated.
However, some caution should be exercised when using targets. First,
setting targets for particular types of contraceptives can provide an
incentive for the agent to emphasize that method, undermining the
provision of information and client choice. Second, applying the same
targets to all agents may not be fair. It does not allow for the
differences in the client populations which agents are serving.
Religion, ethnicity, age, education and other demographic variables
can all have an impact on acceptance of family planning which is quite
separate from agent performance. Therefore, some thought should be
given to individualizing targets so as to encourage rather than
discourage agents working in more difficult settings.

To set appropriate targets, it is advisable to review the past experience of other programs. People who know the characteristics of
particular communities and the agents themselves should be involved
in the target-setting process. Finally, the program staff should, if
necessary, be willing to modify targets which have been established.

Forms

The physical design of forms used for data collection is a crucial
element of an MIS. It is closely correlated with compliance and accuracy. Forms must be easy to carry, clear, uncluttered and quick to use.
When possible, the forms should be designed so that data only needs
to be entered once. This increases compliance by minimizing the staff
time required to complete the forms, and decreases error due to
mistakes made in transcription. In addition, a system of built-in feedback or results can be provided. Forms can be made easier to use by
using color-coding and graphics. Often these features are expensive,
and their benefits and costs must be carefully considered. For non-
literate CBD agents or clients, forms using pictures and simple counts
can be used.

The next case study, Dealing with Data, describes FPAM's Evaluation
Unit, and the process it goes through in designing a management information system for the community-based distribution program. The
cases which follow illustrate this system in use from the perspective of
the organization's central Evaluation Unit, the supervisors, and the
agents. You will be asked to identify strengths and limitations of this
system, and suggest modifications which can make it more useful. Use
the ideas you have just read about to assist you.

CASE 4:   DEALING WITH DATA

(The following case is divided into two parts.)

Case Learning Points

- Identify information needed by staff at different levels of the CBD program, and how this relates to their job performance. Understand how this information can be used to improve program management.

- Understand how to analyze and critique an existing information system.

- Identify the organizational problems in the evaluation department that led to the situation described in the case. Identify some possible solutions.

A) Case Study: Dealing With Data (I)

Four years earlier, as part of FPAM's organizational restructuring, the board of directors decided to remove the program evaluation responsibility from the program managers by broadening the role of the statistical officer. Mr. William Alphonse was hired for this new position and given the title of Evaluation Officer. In addition to evaluation, he was responsible for developing an ongoing management information system. He was also assigned to network with other agencies interested in population policy and to provide support for government policy decision making.

The position was very attractive and competition had been intense. Ten candidates were interviewed by the FPAM board of directors. Although he had had no previous experience in family planning, Mr. Alphonse's undergraduate and graduate training in demography and evaluation got him the job.

During his first year at FPAM, Mr. Alphonse spent the majority of his time on matters related to population policy: fact finding, research, and drafting policy statements. He was so successful at this that he was asked by the government to be a member of the Momonboro delegation to the International Conference on Population in Mexico City. When he wasn't working on policy issues, he was busy helping the information, education and communication officer pre-test educational materials, making supervisory visits, and performing interim evaluations of project personnel with the National Program Coordinator.

In his second year at FPAM, Mr. Alphonse was called into Mrs. Tyler's office. During their meeting, she asked him to help her prepare the management information system component of the CBD project proposal. Over the next several months, Mr. Alphonse consulted the project documents and examined the general project activities and objectives, the project organizational chart (see page 44), and the job descriptions for the staff to be hired. Mr. Alphonse identified the levels in the system and developed a list of information that he thought was needed for managing the program effectively at each level.

Study Questions

1. Identify the key management levels in the CBD project and describe the types of decisions and responsibility for each level.

2. Make a list of the information you think needs to be collected at each management level.

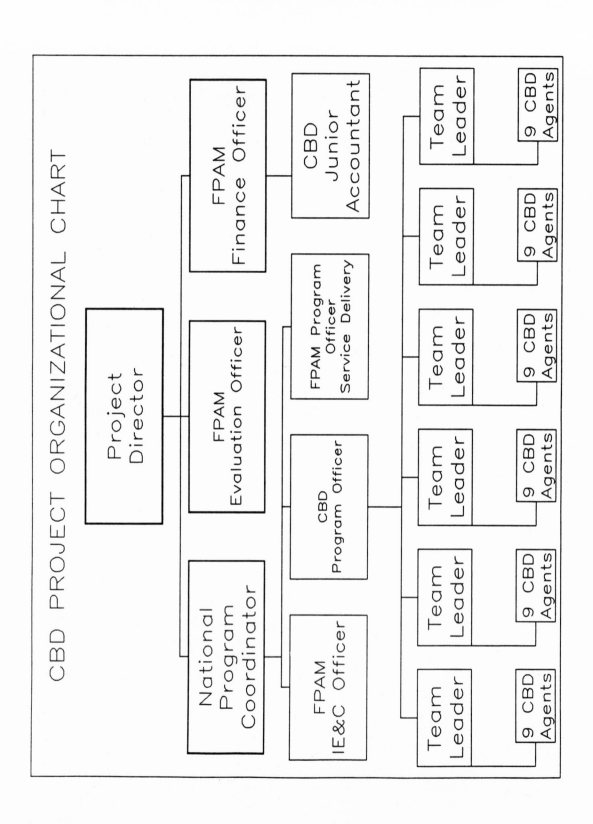

CBD PROJECT ORGANIZATIONAL CHART

B) Case Analysis: Dealing with Data (I)

While there are a number of levels of responsibility and decision-making in the program, we will focus on three: the distributor, the team leader, and the program officer. Based on the project design, each position entails a number of different functions for which information will be necessary. The list below contains some of the important ones. You may have identified others.

Distributor

The distributor is responsible for "front-line management" of the program. She or he will be responsible for contacting, educating and recruiting clients, helping them to determine an appropriate contraceptive method, supplying them with contraceptives, monitoring whether they are used, and following up with those who do not return for supplies. The agent will also refer to the clinic people who wish to use clinical methods or have medical problems. She or he will also need to keep track of money received, and how many contacts and referrals have been made.

Information collected at the distributor level should include:

- Basic client characteristics (name/age/sex/address)
- Type and quantity of contraceptive distributed to each client
- Money collected and outstanding bills
- Information and education contacts made
- Referrals by method
- Dropouts and reason for discontinuation

Most of this information focuses on the individual client. For the distributor to be able to evaluate her or his own performance, she or he also needs to have some aggregate information on the overall numbers she or he has been responsible for in these categories. It may be useful for the distributor to calculate some simple ratios, such as acceptors/client contact, and number of successful referrals, i.e. those who actually visit the clinic.

Team Leader

The team leader serves as a community-based intermediary between the distributor and the program staff based at headquarters. She or he is responsible for immediate supervision of distributors, and verification of their activities. In addition, the team leader might be responsible for recruiting and training distributors.

At the team leader level, the following information should be collected:

- Number of contacts per distributor
- Number of new clients per distributor
- Number of active users per distributor
- Number of effective referrals per distributor
- Number of dropouts per distributor
- Money collected and outstanding per distributor
- Number of distributors recruited
- Number of distributors trained

These data could be used as performance indicators to compare the performance of distributors and to uncover the reasons for success which could perhaps be replicated. The team leader will also want to have a record of the performance of her or his team as a whole, and perhaps to compare this with the record of other teams.

CBD Program Officer

The CBD program officer is responsible for monitoring the program and for supervising the team leaders. This person is the primary link between the agents and the broader program. At this level, the information from the team leaders should be compiled for supervision, monitoring the performance of the team leaders, and for reporting the progress of the whole program to the office. For the purposes of resupply and remuneration, information on income generated and commodities supplied is also necessary.

In addition to the above, the program officer will need to know:

- Usage of different commodities for resupply
- Performance indicators (see above)
- Comparative data between agents and teams

These data should be reported both UPWARD to the project director, and DOWNWARD to the team leaders and agents through monthly feedback to each team on their performance, ranking them in comparison with other groups. Information about program performance should also be shared periodically with the community leaders.

Systems and forms for gathering and transmitting this information will need to be incorporated in the management information system (MIS). The next case will discuss the process of planning the MIS, and some broader issues related to managing the evaluation unit in FPAM.

A) Case Study: Dealing With Data (II)

FPAM's community-based distribution project had received final approval for funding in November of the previous year. However, detailed plans for implementing the management information system were not begun until a training workshop held the following May. The training consultants brought several MIS models from other countries with them. The staff felt that none of the reporting systems seemed particularly relevant to Momonboro, and therefore decided to design and develop their own reporting forms.

Although they did not have time to complete the entire MIS system, they designed the CBD agent record, the team leader's monthly report form, and the CBD program officer's monthly report form (pages 49-51). Overall, Mr. Alphonse was extremely pleased with the progress that had been made. He felt that having the input and participation of the group would be of great help when it came time to train the team leaders and distributors in using the system.

Shortly after the workshop, the community distributors were trained (see Annex 4 for their training curriculum), and in July they began work in their communities. Unfortunately, Mr. Alphonse had been very busy. He had been out of the country studying evaluation systems in neighboring countries for two months. Immediately after he returned, he spent one month traveling up-country interviewing personnel for the annual evaluation of supervisory visits.

When he returned to the office, Mr. Alphonse turned his attention to the data collected by the CBD program, but found that the information had not yet reached his office. He then focused on the interim evaluation that he was to develop to assess the first six months of project activity.

Mr. Alphonse was bothered by the fact that no plans had been made in the initial project design to permit him direct access to the data. He felt that this would make it difficult for him to provide effective support to the project, or to develop the reports outlined in the project paper.

Mr. Alphonse did not object to the information going to the CBD program officer and financial officer. He had accompanied them on supervisory visits and had seen them using the information to monitor the program in the field. However, he thought that it might be better if his office could get the data first, and then analyze and present it to them. This required some time and expertise, and he felt he could assist the program officer with this work. He knew that the community leaders were not getting the quarterly reports that they had been promised, but only summaries of raw data. A microcomputer and an assistant would help him be of real assistance to the CBD program officer.

There was another issue troubling Mr. Alphonse. He hadn't had the time to develop the management reporting system for the CBD project that had been planned in the project paper. Because he had been so busy he hadn't had time to design a basic set of management reports. Tomorrow, if the Executive Director and the rest of the staff would just leave him in peace, he would begin to work it out.

Study Questions

1. Describe the existing information system for the CBD program. What are the advantages and disadvantages of the current system?

2. Identify some of the problems facing Mr. Alphonse in his role as the Evaluation Officer.

Data Collection Form for CBD Agent

Name of CBD Agent: _____   Location: _____   Zone: _____

Date of 1st CBD Service	Client Information					Reg. No.	Contraceptives Distributed												Referrals Made							Side Eff		Month	
	Name & Address	Age	Sex	Educ	No. of Live Children		Pills			Crm/Paste			Foam/Tblts			Condoms			Medical Checkup			Steriliz			NF		No. of Ref
							NA	CA	Qty	NA	CA	Qty	NA	CA	Qty	NA	CA	Qty	Pills	IUD	Injec	M	F	Eff	P		

No. of Contacts Made _____

Key of Contraceptives Distributed
NA = New Acceptor
CA = Continuing Acceptor
Qty = Quantity
Crm = Spermicidal Cream
Tblts = Spermicidal Tablets

Key of Pills Distributed (To fill in)
Noriday = NRD   Microgynon = MCRG
Femenal = FEM   Nordette = NDL
Low Femenal = L/FEM   Microlute = MCL
Ovral = OV   Eugynon = EUG

Key of Dropouts
Pregnancy = PREG
Side Effects = SE
Migration = MIG
Natural Family Planning = NFP

Team Leader's Monthly Report Form

Name of Team Leader: _____   Area: _____   Reporting Period: _____

Name of Agent	Zone	Contraceptives Distributed														Effective Referrals				Sterilization		Medic Check	Side Effe	Drop Outs			
		Pills			Crm/Paste			Foam/Tblts			Condoms				Pills	IUD	Inj		M	F			NFP	Spouse	Preg	
		Con	NA	CA	Qty	NA	CA	Qty	NA	CA	Qty	NA	CA	Qty												

Totals

Key

Zon = Zone	M = Male
Con = Number of Contacts	F = Female
NA = New Acceptors	Medic Check = Medical Check-up
CA = Continuing Acceptors	NFP = Natural Family Planning
Qty = Quantity	Spouse = Spouse's Objection
Crm = Spermicidal Cream	Preg = Pregnant
Tblts = Spermicidal Tablets	
Inj = Injectables (Depo Provera)	

Program Officer's Monthly Report Form

Monthly/Quarterly Report for period starting _____July 1_____ and ending _____July 31_____

SERVICE DELIVERY	Placatte	Nukrutown	East Middleton	Clear–water	Royalton	TOTALS
1. No of Distributors Reporting	19	8	10	10	7	54
2. New Acceptors						
pill	208	69	151	187	64	679
condom	237	15	104	140	42	538
foam	82	27	26	71	28	234
foam tablets	64	47	41	98	24	274
IUD						
injectables						
other						
3. Referrals						
pill						
IUD						
injectables						
sterilization						
side effects						
FP check up	4					4
other health problems	27					27
4. Active Users						
new clients	591	158	322	496	158	1725
continuing acceptors *	347	155	111	144	56	813
5. Reasons for Dropout						
husband/relative						
method side effect						
gone away/death						
pregnancy/disease						
rumors						
other						

* Continuing Acceptors: Figures indicate continuing acceptors from previous usage of Contraceptive Methods form.

B) Case Analysis: Dealing with Data (II)

The two parts of this case deal with several issues related to program evaluation and management information systems.

The Information System

The process of establishing the MIS is an important one. In Dealing With Data (I), Mr. Alphonse approached the initial conceptualization of the MIS methodically by reviewing the program material. He then outlined information which he thought would be useful in managing the program.

When it came time to actually design and implement the MIS, he asked for the input and participation of the users. They designed draft forms for the agent, the team leader, and the program officer. While this demonstrates initiative, it is not without problems.

The CBD form seems to contain a lot of useful information, but not in a very clear format. The CBD agent probably will not refer back to this form to evaluate her or his own performance. Furthermore, it does not readily supply the information necessary for the team leader's report.

The team leader's report has some similar drawbacks, as does the program officer's report. As we will see in the next two cases, the format and information contained in these two reports is not always useful to the users.

Another problem is how the information system is organized. The data does not seem to move systematically. While, as Mr. Alphonse acknowledges, it is useful for the financial manager and the program officer to have access to the information, he finds himself physically removed from the data. This prevents him from using the information for his evaluation reports, and from making it more useful to the rest of the staff through analysis. Furthermore, he is not getting the data back into the community as he promised.

The Evaluation Unit

In the broader sense, Mr. Alphonse's job is complicated by the fact that he does not seem to have a clearly defined role in the organization. As mentioned in the background notes for this section, separating evaluation from program activities may have benefits, but it also creates some problems. While the evaluation officer may have the skills, the time, and an objective perspective, she or he may be viewed as somewhat threatening by the program managers. This may explain why, as mentioned above, the data are not reaching her or his office. The Evaluation Officer's role needs to be very carefully defined for the program staff to maximize effectiveness and minimize friction.

An additional problem is that Mr. Alphonse has been so overloaded with other tasks that he has not had time to address the CBD program. This is a frequent management problem where external demands are so extensive that someone is unable to carry out all of their responsibilities.

These organizational problems and Mr. Alphonse's role need to be addressed by senior management. The next cases will demonstrate how the MIS is working, or not working, at the lower levels of the CBD program.

CASE 5:   THE JEFFERSONVILLE SUPERVISORY MEETING

Case Learning Points

- Understand how targets and specific indicators can be used to evaluate and improve performance.

- Understand how to assess the feasibility of changing or adding targets or indicators to a program.

- Understand how to present information so that it is useful and can have a positive impact on program performance.

A) Case Study: The Jeffersonville Supervisory Meeting

At exactly two o'clock in the afternoon, four FPAM staff members walked out of the central office and piled into the car. Betty Amaya, the CBD program officer, Ester Elgazan, the Project Officer for Service Delivery, Louis Armstrong, the CBD Junior Accountant, and William Alphonse the Evaluation Officer, were headed for Jeffersonville to conduct their monthly supervisory meeting.

Arriving at the town hall, they were greeted by a large number of community distributors and local men. The community was holding a contest in the hall that afternoon, so another location had to be found for the supervisory meeting. After some initial confusion, the team leader quickly arranged for the use of a nearby school. The entire group moved down the street to the dusty, hot, single room school house. Several of the distributors rearranged the benches and swept out the dust while the group set up for the meeting.

The Jeffersonville supervisory meeting covered three urban communities: Bossa, Slipyaw, and Jeffersonville itself. Because of the size of the area, there were three teams of ten distributors. Each team had its own team leader. The distributors here appeared relatively well dressed, poised, and self-confident. Most were high school graduates, although only a few worked at other jobs. The Jeffersonville team leader was a university student, Mr. Somatta. The team leaders from Slipyaw and Bossa were older women from these communities, Mrs. Ababa and Mrs. Entewe.

Each of the distributors wore a cloth badge stenciled with red letters "CBD Distributor FPAM" pinned to their shirt. Each carried a big black leather bag with 'FPAM' stenciled in white letters on the side. Perhaps because of the change of venue, several of the distributors were absent and the rest of the group waited on the benches fanning themselves in the heat. To save time, Mr. Armstrong agreed with Mrs. Elgazan that they should pass around the attendance roster. He asked the distributors to mark the quantity of supplies they needed next to their names. In this way he would be able to prepare each supply order before the end of the meeting.

Mr. Somatta sent one of the distributors back to the town hall to pin a note on the door informing the latecomers of the new meeting place. By the time he had returned, several more distributors had arrived and Mrs. Elgazan passed out the agenda for the meeting. One agent volunteered to say the opening prayer and the meeting began.

Mrs. Elgazan opened the session by asking if any of the distributors had had problems since their last meeting. Seravia was the first to raise her hand and stand. She recounted the story of an adolescent girl on the pill who was being advised to discontinue it by her aunt. "What can I do about this?" she asked.

Rather than respond herself, Mrs. Elgazan asked if anybody in the group had any suggestions for Seravia. Mr. Johnson volunteered, "Why don't you talk to the aunt? I would try to convince the aunt about the importance of family planning. Then maybe she will get off of her niece's back."

Another distributor spoke up and said, "I agree with Mr. Johnson. When you promote family planning you need to involve everyone in the family, not just the person who uses it. Last month one of my clients wanted to stop using the pill because her nine-month-old son had just died of measles. She already had five children and was in poor health herself. But her husband wanted another baby and was pressing her to stop using the pill. As a man, it was easy for me to go to the husband and convince him to allow his wife to defer pregnancy so that she could improve her own health and have a healthier baby at a later date."

Noticing that three distributors were missing, Mrs. Elgazan asked where they were. Mrs. Ebewe volunteered that one was not able to come because of another commitment. She had been out to check on the other two, she said, and one was sick and not very interested in the work, and the other had said that she wanted to quit.

Mrs. Amaya broke in, holding up the team leaders summary sheet that she had just received. "How many contacts are you supposed to make a month?" she asked the agents.

"Sixty," said one of the agents.

"That's right," she said. "And out of those sixty, how many new acceptors on the average should you recruit?"

There was silence for a while, and then someone volunteered, "Six."

"Good," said Mrs. Amaya. "But look at this data. Here we have over 2600 contacts and only eighty-seven new acceptors. What have you all been doing, counting every person you shake hands with? Maybe you're not spending enough time with the clients. Some of you have very low acceptor rates. In fact two of the agents missing today didn't get a single acceptor last month. What are you doing about this?" she asked Mrs. Ebewe.

"To be honest," she answered, "I've given up on them."

"But that means no one is serving their areas. You've got to reassign areas when you have a problem like this."

"But I didn't notice it until you pointed it out just now. It's hard to tell what's going on from the form I fill out for you."

"OK," Mrs. Amaya said. "We'll go over that next week together." She put the form down and turned the meeting over to the financial officer, Mr. Armstrong.

After the meeting, Mrs. Amaya thought about the problem of targets. She wondered if the targets that she was using were good ones. She felt that she could be doing much more to help the team leaders. If she had a chance to do some analysis of the data she was getting on the team leaders summary sheet, she could give them some simple feedback on their agents and their team's performance.

Study Questions

1. How useful are the targets that Mrs. Amaya is using?

2. Can you think of other targets that might help improve agent performance? If some of these targets require more information, how could you get it? Would it be worth it?

3. What suggestions would you make to Mrs. Amaya to improve feedback to the team leader about the performance of the team and to agents about their performance?

B) Case Analysis: The Jeffersonville Supervisory Meeting

This case identifies some problems in agent performance and in the information system which is being used to evaluate it.

There are a few agents who are doing poorly, and need to be assisted or replaced. Problems like this are to be expected of any new program. The key is to identify the problems early on, and attempt to resolve them quickly.

Usefulness of Targets

A great deal of effort seems to be focused on contacts, and not enough on new acceptors. Mrs. Amaya is rightfully concerned about the contact/acceptor ratio. This may be a result of the targets and the management information system. Emphasizing the number of contacts could be encouraging the agents to inflate the numbers of contacts to make the data look good. Yet their payment is linked primarily to contraceptive sales, not contacts, so there is certainly no financial reward for doing this.

The real problem lies in the number of new acceptors. For each agent the target is set at six new acceptors per month. Therefore, eighty-seven acceptors for three teams of nine agents is clearly substandard. This is the true target of the program, and if it is not being reached, changes should be made. It may require that more time be spent with each contact, or more visits made to each one.

There could be several explanations for the agents' substandard performance. One is that the agents are not working effectively or efficiently. An alternative is that the target is set too high. This is difficult to ascertain, but certainly comparisons across districts and between agents can provide some useful information. As discussed in the background notes for this section, the supervisors must be careful not to rely solely on raw numbers. Targets should be individualized to allow for demographic variation. It would be unfair to compare the statistics, for example, of an agent working in the university quarter to an agent working in a Moslem neighborhood. While allowances must be made for variation, the data itself is very important. Getting this information may encourage the senior staff to try new strategies in difficult areas.

Other Potential Targets

With regard to setting specific targets, a number of other possible indicators could be used. The dropout rate and the length of active use are important, relevant performance measures, and if they are formalized as targets, an additional incentive is introduced to achieve them. Perhaps acceptors should be targeted for specific lengths of time, depending on their reproductive intentions. In addition, performance measures based on ratios would provide information about the effectiveness of certain client activities. This would be useful for both the agents and the supervisors. A measure such as number of acceptors per contact could be calculated from the information already being collected.

Integrating additional targets and performance indicators into the program would require collecting more information. Average length of contraception, agent time spent in various activities, and dropout rates would all require that additional data be compiled by the agent. An increase in resources would be needed to collect the additional information, as the MIS forms would need to be modified and printed, the distributors would need to be retrained, and more time would be spent collecting and recording the additional information. More time would also be required at the central and supervisory levels to process and use the data.

These costs may seem significant at first, but once this "investment" is made, and the indicators are integrated into the system, the costs to continue to generate this information will be minimal. Because the performance indicators being used at present are too limited, the additional cost of expanding the base of information might be warranted.

If the decision is made to change the data forms, all staff members should be consulted. A hidden danger of the expansion of the information system is that if too much information is collected, it may overwhelm the staff.

Improving Feedback

Mrs. Amaya is also aware of the fact that relevant information needs to be available at the service delivery level. Agents and team leaders need to be able to compare their performance against their targets, as well as against the performance of other CBD workers. This requires the design of a simpler, more appropriate set of forms with a quick turnaround time, and perhaps the use of graphics to demonstrate performance.

Mrs. Amaya has identified a legitimate problem, and should approach the Evaluation Officer, as well as the agents and the team leaders, to help resolve it.

CASE 6:   MR. KRUMAH'S DILEMMA

Case Learning Points

- Understand what information is important to CBD agents, and how they use this information to conduct their work.

- Understand how the design of the MIS system and the data collection form affects the use of information.

- Identify strategies for addressing the problems with the MIS outlined in the previous cases.

A) Case Study: Mr. Krumah's Dilemma

Mr. Krumah sat on the wooden bench in front of his house and watched the children playing football in the street. Tomorrow the CBD team leader was scheduled to visit him to review his record book. Today he planned to bring his records up to date.

Mr. Krumah took out the notebook that he had been given when he became a community distributor. He had carefully drawn a table with the following headings:

> name/address
> age/sex
> acceptor/registration number
> contraceptives by type and quantity
> date of next visit

He examined the information which he had penciled in under each column every time one of his motivational talks had resulted in a client accepting a family planning method. The wooden table where he was working was small, but he had managed to open and spread out both his notebook and the oversized agent record form booklet. He now began the tedious process of transferring the data from his own notebook onto the project record form which the team leader would review.

Mr. Krumah had been a distributor for six months now, and each time he went through this transfer process he felt increasingly irritated. When the team leader came he didn't collect the agent record forms, but only looked at them to summarize the data for his own purposes. What Mr. Krumah found annoying was that he had all the information the team leader needed in his own notebook. Filling out the record form each month was just additional work. He decided that he would take up this issue with Mr. Somatta, the team leader, when he called the following day.

Mr. Somatta arrived in mid-morning. "How are you?" Mr. Somatta asked.

"Fine," said Mr. Krumah. "It's hot. Take a drink?"

"Thank you," said Mr. Somatta as he sat down on the porch within the shade of the tin roof. Mr. Krumah sent a child to get two drinks from the nearby store. "How did it go this month?"

"Fine," Mr. Krumah responded. "I had a good month. I had eighteen new acceptors." He pulled out his notebook and his record forms and handed Mr. Somatta the record book. Taking a deep breath, he said, "There is something that bothers me. Every month I fill out these forms for you but you don't take them." Then, handing Mr. Somatta the notebook, he continued, "This is the book I use to keep track of my clients." Mr. Somatta took the book and looked at the table that Mr. Krumah had devised. "If you took the data that you need out of my notebook, I wouldn't need to fill out the agent record form."

Mr. Somatta studied the two books. "This is excellent," he said. "You have a very organized notebook. But most people don't keep such nice books."

"Maybe you could make an exception for me," Mr. Krumah suggested. "Filling out these forms is really getting tiresome."

"I'll have to give that some thought," Mr. Somatta said. "Why don't you bring it up at the next supervisory meeting?"

"There's something else," Mr. Krumah said. "You know I work as a canvasser for an insurance company part time. The most important thing is to get the money for the premium before the end of the month. If I don't, the subscriber loses his policy and I lose my commission. Family planning is just the same. I need to know the date when the woman needs a new cycle of pills. If I don't see her on time she will get pregnant and I'll lose my fee."

"That's true," agreed Mr. Somatta. "It's extremely helpful to keep track of the date when you need to make a resupply visit." He took a drink and began summarizing the data he needed from Mr. Krumah's record book. He transferred information on new acceptors, continuing acceptors and quantities of contraceptives distributed to his monthly team leader summary form.

Study Questions

1. What information is useful to the CBD agent? How does he use this information?

2. Why did the agent, Mr. Krumah, develop his own record keeping system?

3. Should Mr. Krumah bring the issue up at the supervisory meeting?

4. Should the team leader allow Mr. Krumah to discontinue using the official agent record form?

B) Case Analysis: Mr. Krumah's Dilemma

This case depicts the information system from the perspective of the individual CBD agent. Together with the two preceding cases, we can now identify changes which should be made in the management information system to make it more relevant to all its users.

Information Useful for the Agents

In order to design a management information system which is useful for the distributors, both the method of record-keeping and the specific information contained must be modified. Certainly the schedule for revisits which Mr. Krumah has included must be considered, as well as the distributors' inventory of supplies. At present the agents are left on their own to monitor these two important items. In addition, the current record form is physically too bulky for the distributors to carry around. While Mr. Krumah has designed an effective alternative, completing the forms for the team leader's visit doubles his record-keeping tasks. This increases the possibility of errors, and has become a tedious chore.

Mr. Krumah has identified the problem, and come up with a useful, though burdensome, way of working around it. However, other agents may not be as resourceful, and may therefore have problems keeping track of necessary information. It would be helpful to incorporate this information formally into the system, and to design a form which not only collects data for management, but serves as a useful tool at the distributor level.

Raising the Problems

The team leader suggests that Mr. Krumah bring his problems and suggestions up at the next supervisory meeting. This raises the interesting issue of how to initiate change in the system. It is not clear that this is or should be Mr. Krumah's responsibility. Furthermore, while Mr. Krumah should be given credit for his suggestions, they might be more influential if raised by the team leader. This seems particularly true given the situation described in the previous cases.

Staying with the System

Because the management information process needs to remain systematic, it is doubtful that the team leader will allow Mr. Krumah to stop using the official forms entirely. However, Mr. Krumah has some very constructive suggestions. The important issue is whether or not the problems he has raised and his ideas for modifying the system will be acted upon.

There are problems with the existing management information system at all levels. The team leaders expressed difficulty following individual distributor performance. The supervisors acknowledged that the system was not clear or effective. Finally, even Mr. Alphonse, who is ultimately responsible for designing the system, knows there are problems, both for his own use and at several other levels. It is clear that some modifications and changes should be made.

PART IV   SUPERVISION

Overview

The next case addresses supervision. Supervision is an important
management tool. It can be used to improve staff performance, and to
monitor, identify, and address problems early on. Like planning and
management information systems, supervision occurs at many levels
of an organization. This case deals primarily with the supervision of
community-based distribution agents and team leaders by staff
members from the FPAM central program office.

Supervision can be defined as overseeing the work of others. It has
three primary functions:

1. technical assistance

2. monitoring and evaluation

3. motivation and support of workers

In many programs, the process of supervision is also closely linked to
data collection, logistics, and resupply.

It is important to build a formal system of supervision into a program.
The specific structure of a supervisory system for any program is
determined by a number of factors. These include: the background of
the person being supervised; the complexity of the task; the personal
style of both the supervisor and the worker; the atmosphere of the
organization; and the culture in which the program is operating. When
setting up a supervisory system, all of these elements must be taken
into consideration.

While a supervisor needs to check on and monitor the performance of
workers, she or he should primarily be a supportive problem solver
rather than a critical disciplinarian. It is as important to recognize
good work as it is to notice and correct an inadequate or flawed
performance.

Providing feedback on performance is central to supervision. A
crucial element of this process is that the people being supervised
know what is expected of them. In many programs this is facilitated

by the use of forms and checklists. These can be very helpful in providing some standard measures to judge performance, but they can also be limiting. They can prevent the supervisor from addressing the particular needs of the individuals and the job they are doing. When completed on-site, checklists also tend to reinforce the "policing" function of the supervisor rather than the supporting function.

To effectively provide feedback, the supervisor should involve the employees in the process. The supervisor should create an atmosphere of teamwork. A friendly tone should be set for the meeting, and participation and discussion encouraged. People will feel more comfortable sharing their problems and concerns if they are confident that they will not be punished for raising them.

Supervision can be conducted individually or in groups. When possible, it is desirable to observe employees in the actual settings where they work. Less tangible issues of style and client interaction can be observed and constructively criticized.

Supervision in CBD Programs

Supervision is central to any organization, but it is particularly important in community-based distribution programs. CBD agents may have limited training and experience in the technical aspects of their work, in effectively working in a community, and in reporting and accounting procedures. In many settings, distributors are working in isolation, with little contact with the rest of the program. Furthermore, remuneration for their work is often minimal or sporadic.

Effective supervision of CBD agents can help to address these problems. Supervisory visits can be used to provide clarification and on-going instruction in technical, outreach, and reporting functions. Particularly in isolated areas, supervisors can serve as a link between the distributors and the broader program. The supervisor should convey information both to the distributors and from them. In a situation where remuneration is limited, supervisory visits can be an important source of motivation.

In many community-based distribution programs, the distance separating distributors means that reliable transportation and a significant amount of staff time are required to supervise agents individually. Supervision of CBD agents is therefore often done in groups, where both the supervisor and the distributors meet at a central location to review their work. This type of supervision is useful in enabling distributors to share common experiences and to learn from one another. This can be beneficial in CBD programs where there is usually little other chance for interaction between agents. It is important, however, for the supervisor to be aware of the performance and the special needs of individuals within the group. Participation and, when necessary, individual discussions must be included.

The intensity and frequency of supervisory visits will vary considerably between programs, depending on transportation, how long the program has been in operation, and the tasks performed by the supervisor during the visit. In a new program, frequent supervision is important. When both the program and staff are more established and experienced, supervisory visits or activities can be conducted less often. It is important to schedule visits in advance and plan for a realistic schedule of visits. While there are no absolute guidelines, a general rule is to schedule supervisory visits or activities as frequently as possible, at least every three months.

Checklists and forms which quantify work can often be used to facilitate the monitoring function. As discussed in the previous section on management information systems, supervisors are often also responsible for relaying performance and health data to the next level of the system. If a supervisor is responsible for reviewing and compiling forms which the distributor has completed, it is important to review them on-site so that any problems can be corrected.

It is vital to remember that supervision is a **process** which helps the organization to achieve its objectives. While effective supervision is an important element in a program, remember that its primary function is to improve the performance of the workers and, through them, the program.

CASE 7:   ROYALTON SUPERVISORY MEETING

Case Learning Points

- Identify and understand the components of effective supervision.

- Understand how a supervisor can use information and specific targets to improve distributor performance.

A) Case Study: The Royalton Monthly Supervisory Meeting

Mrs. Betty Amaya, the Program Officer for the Community-Based Distribution project, had just returned from six weeks of training in California. Even though she was tired from her trip, she was eager to return to work. Mrs. Amaya had a special relationship with this team of community distributors. She barely had time to get out of the car before she was embraced by the distributors waiting at the front door of Redemption Hospital.

With the exception of two men, the community distributors in this group were all young women from Royalton, an outlying area of Placatte. As they crowded in front of the car waiting to welcome her, Mrs. Amaya could see the hard life of the city written on their youthful, anxious faces. Like those in Jeffersonville, pinned to each of their shirts was a cloth badge stenciled with the red letters 'CBD Distributor FPAM.'

The distributors rearranged the clinic benches into a horseshoe shape while Mrs. Amaya and Miss Elgazan, the Program Officer for Service Delivery, paid a quick visit to Dr. Nimpson, the clinic medical director. When they returned, Miss Elgazan passed out the agenda for the meeting.

The team leader, Mr. Bele, was quick to point out that most of the distributors were present, and explained the absence of three distributors. He noted that Philippa would be a little late because she had to walk from work, that Hetty was ill, and that Agatha had unfortunately confused the date of the meeting and made other plans. Miss Elgazan briefly inquired about this as she had sent the regular monthly announcement notifying the team leaders of the schedule of supervisory visits at the beginning of the month, a full ten days before the first supervisory visit was scheduled. Helen then asked that someone approve the agenda and several distributors nodded their accord.

The meeting was officially opened when Miss Elgazan asked one of the distributors to say a short prayer. She then invited the team leader to make some opening remarks. Mr. Bele, a local government official, had been chosen by the group of agents from Royalton as their team leader. He divided his time between the commissioner's office and the project. He cleared his throat and welcomed the group to the meeting.

Miss Elgazan who had now placed herself in a chair facing the group, cried out, "Are you with me?" in a rising tone.

"We're with you!" came the response loudly and in unison.

"Are you the best CBD agents?" Miss Elgazan cried again.

"We're the BEST!" they cried even louder.

"OK," Miss Elgazan said, and immediately held up a blue card. "What's this?" she asked, pointing to the card and displaying it to the group.

"A referral card," came the response from several of the distributors.

"Has anyone been selling this card?" Miss Elgazan asked, and then waited while the group looked on in silence. After a short while she said, "Good. Nobody on this team has been selling them. But elsewhere, it's come to my attention that these cards are being sold for one momambi. These are referral cards and you are right. They are not to be sold. The pink cards which the client receives when she registers at the clinic cost one momambi, and you know that it would be unfair for a client to purchase two cards." She put the referral card back in her folder and placed the folder on her lap. She paused a moment and then, addressing the group collectively said, "It's time to share with each other the problems you've had since our last meeting."

The eight distributors, which now included the late arrival, remained silent, fidgeting nervously and looking anxiously at each other. Miss Elgazan waited, watching and smiling. After some time she said, "Come on now. You all know the importance of discussing our problems together."

She paused a moment, and then continued. "Remember that tall doctor who was here last month? Remember the discussion we had about problems you'd had? Well, that discussion convinced us to get those calculators that you said you needed." She waited again, and then looked at Zelda. "How about you, Zelda, surely you've had some problem in the last month."

Zelda broke the silence by recounting the story of a woman she had met while at the house of one of her clients whom she was resupplying with a month's cycle of pills. Zelda described how the woman had become furious with her, saying that her preaching family planning was an evil lie. "I've taken the pill," she said, "and it didn't work. I got pregnant. You and your family planning organization want us to believe in lies."

Mrs. Amaya, sitting on the bench beside her, asked Zelda gently, "And what did you say?"

"I kept asking her how she was taking the pill, and where she had gotten it. She had bought them at a pharmacy for M4.50 and had never been properly instructed on how to take them."

"Does everybody understand," Mrs. Amaya asked, "what happened here? The family planning program and you are being blamed for something that you didn't do. Who is responsible for this?"

"It's the pharmacist," one of the distributors said. "They never instruct the people how to use the pills."

"That's so important." Mrs. Amaya said. "And what did you tell her?"

"I kept telling her how to take the pill properly," Zelda said. "I told her if she had taken it properly she wouldn't have gotten pregnant. And finally she seemed to believe me. I said I would come back after the baby was born."

"You really held your ground," Mrs. Amaya said. "You have confidence in yourself and you have to take the time if you are going to get the truth out. That was good work."

Robert, one of the two male distributors, spoke up immediately. "I don't know what to tell people about IUDs. People say that they don't work."

Miss Elgazan broke in. "First of all," she said, "when it comes to IUDs remember that your only responsibility is to refer people who want one or who are having problems with one to the clinic."

"Yes, I know that," Robert said. "But people are always asking me. What should I tell them?"

"You can explain to them that IUDs do work about nine out of ten times, but because a doctor must insert the IUD it is better to come to the clinic and have the doctor explain how it works and what the risks and side-effects are. Because the IUD works continuously once it is inserted it is a good method for women who have children and want to space their next pregnancy."

Mrs. Amaya then asked, "How many of you know how many new acceptors you had last month?"

Several distributors volunteered some numbers, "A hundred." "Seventy-six." "Eighty-five."

Mrs. Amaya looked puzzled. "I think you are thinking of continuing users, who have been using family planning for a while," she said. "New acceptors are new people who have never used birth control before, who have started using it just this month."

After some confusion several distributors gave new numbers. "Twenty." "Four." "Thirteen." "Twenty-nine."

"This is a question that we should be able to answer," said Miss Elgazan. "You need to understand the meaning of these terms. Remember, our target for new acceptors is six per month for each CBD agent. If you know what your targets are, it will help you to evaluate your own performance."

Miss Elgazan then held up the data summary sheets that she had received from the team leader for the past month. "We get these sheets from all the team leaders at the end of the month and some of them are very messy because of crossouts. Look here. How can we read this one?" she said, putting a finger on a crossed-out number in a box. "Would the distributors try to be neat, and the team leaders, too? We all need to be able to read these reports."

Mr. Armstrong, the project financial officer who had been sitting to the side during the discussion, broke in. "I need to make a point about the receipts that you are filling out when you sell products. The receipts I've been getting aren't in order. They go from October 29th, to the 30th, to the 5th. That's not right, is it?" He laughed, and several of the distributors joined in. "Date the receipt on the day that you get the money, not on the day you give out the product. Remember that," he said. "OK, now it's time to collect the reports and money and distribute supplies."

Suddenly everyone was in motion at the different stations that had been set up. When this was finished the distributors returned to their seats. Mrs. Amaya smiled and said "I've been reviewing the reports and noticed that things seem to be going much better. Sales are picking up. Anybody have an explanation?"

"It's better now because we've visited more than once," Vesta said. "They know who we are. We have our badges and they know that we are family planning. Now they let us in."

This seemed like a good time to end the meeting. Miss Elgazan thanked the group and asked someone to say the closing prayer.

Back in the car on the way to the office, Mrs. Amaya leaned back, stretched her arms, and said to Miss Elgazan, "It's great to be home." Then, as an afterthought, she added, "Ester, let's you and I work together on the self-evaluation system."

Study Questions

1. Describe the supervisory style used by Mrs. Amaya and Miss Elgazan. What techniques do they use to encourage participation? How do they take corrective action? What techniques do they use to improve distributor performance?

2. How does a sense of mission help an organization accomplish its goals? How do Mrs. Amaya and Miss Elgazan convey this sense of mission to the agents and team leaders?

3. How would you further develop and implement a self-evaluation system for the distributors?

B) Case Analysis: The Royalton Supervisory Meeting

A great deal about supervision can be learned by analyzing Miss Elgazan's and Mrs. Amaya's actions at this meeting. First of all, the tone they set for the meeting is both official and relaxed. It is clear from their reception that the distributors both like and respect them.

The supervisors are very organized. An agenda is circulated, and while it really contains nothing new, it makes the meeting more official. Attendance is taken, and efforts are made to uncover the reasons for absenteeism. It is clear that everyone is expected to be present. An announcement of the dates of all the monthly supervisory meetings was distributed to all CBD agents in the project. In this way they know well in advance about the meeting times, and can plan ahead to attend. Attention to detail is important if a program is to run smoothly.

Miss Elgazan involves the agents very early in the meeting. The prayer is given by one of the agents, and then the meeting is turned over to the team leader, thereby acknowledging his role. Miss Elgazan quickly moves on to discuss the problem of selling cards. In a non-accusatory, informative manner, she lets it be known that they are not to be sold.

Next she gets the agents to share their experiences. This is the most important part of the meeting. Refusing to accept the inevitable nervous silence, Miss Elgazan coaxes the agents to express themselves. Her ability to provide direction and encouragement from her agents' own experience is an important supervisory skill.

A sense of mission and involvement with the broader project is very important to motivate the agents. The case contains a number of examples of how this can be done. It is highlighted by the chant which starts the meeting. This gives a real sense of belonging to a team. The CBD agents are very goal-oriented and committed in their efforts to distribute contraceptives.

The issue of designing an effective system of self-evaluation for the agents presents an interesting problem which has already been touched on in the previous cases.

There is obviously some misunderstanding about the categories of contacts and acceptors. Agents should look at both their contacts and their clients, and the relationship between the two. Numbers of contacts tend to be inflated because of group encounters. The agents should be looking more closely at factors related to successful contacts, for example, those who become acceptors. Some issues they should think about include: how much time is spent in encounters; how that time is spent; how they are followed up; and which people are most likely to become family planning acceptors.

Finally, the length of contraceptive use for acceptors should be examined. A program with a high number of acceptors but also a high number of dropouts may initially look more successful than a program with fewer acceptors who continue to use family planning for a long time. Overall, however, a program with a high dropout rate is much less successful. This is an issue that Mr. Alphonse and the project management need to work out with the supervisors and the agents.

PART V   COMPENSATION AND PRICING

Overview

Pricing and charging for contraceptives raise a number of sensitive issues. A common notion often prevails that people will not pay for contraceptives, and that governments should provide health services, including family planning, free of charge. With the deepening financial pressures on the governments of many developing countries, free health care systems are often unrealistic and impossible to sustain. In addition, in many places free goods are perceived as inferior, and several recent studies have demonstrated that even poor people want to pay for services. Moreover, an organization like FPAM can use revenues from the sale of donated commodities to support self-sustaining programs which would otherwise be impossible to maintain.

In pricing contraceptives, however, it is important that they remain affordable for the poor, otherwise the community distribution program will exclude those it is targeted to reach. Even the most reasonable price will still exclude some people, and an alternative strategy for providing services and supplies to those who cannot afford to pay should be considered in any system.

Contraceptive Pricing and Agent Compensation

In many programs, the pricing of contraceptives is closely linked to the compensation provided to distribution agents. In most community-based distribution programs, agents are paid, at least in part, by receiving a percentage of the revenue generated by their sales. If the price is set too low, the agents will not be adequately compensated for their work and their motivation will decline.

While some CBD programs have successfully relied on volunteers, most provide compensation in some form. As mentioned above, most have employed a commission system. In some programs, agents have been paid a set salary.

Each system has advantages and drawbacks. Providing distributors with a regular salary offers them income security and compensates all distributors equally. A fixed salary also makes it easier to attract applicants to the program. Unfortunately, this system provides little material incentive for the agents to do their work effectively. It gives the program little control over the quality of the distributor's work or performance.

Using a straight commission, where distributors are paid based only on their sales, provides incentives for productivity, but not for quality. It does not give the distributor a secure and regular income, and would therefore most likely preclude the employment of full-time distributors. There is no guarantee that, even if distributors work hard, they will derive any income from their activities. This is particularly difficult when one must account for extremely different levels of acceptance determined by demographic and cultural variation across neighborhoods or areas.

A straight commission system produces financial data which are directly correlated with program success. Because the goal is to distribute contraceptives, sales represent project outputs. The agents' 50 percent commission means that their motivation and performance is driven primarily by sales, which in turn drives the project.

However, this analysis is not entirely complete or correct. First, as discussed above, some potential clients may not be able to afford to pay for contraceptives. More importantly, sales of commodities are measures of program activity and may not exactly correspond with the project's goals and objectives (for example, providing good services, client compliance, effective child spacing, and population stabilization).

Some programs use bonus systems of awards and prizes for individual agents or teams. These are often used in an attempt to incorporate "qualitative" measures, such as interaction with clients, community involvement, effort, and cooperation, into agent remuneration. Though they are difficult to measure, these are important program components. There is increasing evidence that both acceptor rates and length of contraception improve when clients are able to choose freely between methods, and feel they are being treated respectfully.

The next case addresses these issues, and discusses the solutions to the problems of compensation, quality and pricing that FPAM devised.

CASE 8: THE SALES FORCE

Case Learning Points

- Identify the major issues surrounding the use of different types of financial incentives to motivate community-based distributors.

- Understand how to use sales and financial information to monitor and reward performance.

A) Case Study: The Sales Force

Kokie Tyler knew about money and how to manage it. In her previous job with the Ministry of Finance, she had reorganized the payroll system for government agencies. In developing the CBD program, she was committed to incorporating financial incentives for the distributors. In early discussions with donors and project staff she had considered paying the distributors a monthly salary. However, the funding agency was interested in encouraging the project to become self-supporting, and did not find this acceptable. A new approach was called for and several were suggested, including a self-sustaining income generation scheme. However, Mrs. Tyler resisted this idea, questioning its feasibility in Momonboro.

In conversation with the donors, Mrs. Tyler argued that the sale of contraceptives was also problematic. FPAM had little experience in this area. Even if the products could be sold, she felt uncertain as to whether they could generate sufficient funds to provide adequate remuneration to the distributors.

At the same time, however, experience from two small FPAM pilot projects indicated that selling contraceptives improved acceptor rates. Free pills were viewed as being "dumped" into Momonboro because of their poor quality. This led Mrs. Tyler to decide to try selling contraceptives in the CBD program. Given her uncertainty about the amount of money this would generate, she decided upon a dual reimbursement system. Each distributor would be provided with twenty momambi a month as a "base salary." In addition, they would get a commission of 50 percent of the total revenue from contraceptives sales. Because of the team leaders' added responsibilities, their base salary would be double that of the distributors.

Mrs. Tyler called a meeting of all the distributors to ask how they felt about a sales commission or a salary. While excited about the possibility of receiving a 50 percent commission on sales of pills, foam and condoms, they were worried because this system would require them to manage the money they collected. Mrs. Tyler assured them that this would not be a problem, and that a simple financial control system could be put into place.

To price the contraceptives, Mrs. Tyler decided to use the same rates that had been used in a previous FPAM Project. The prices were:

Type of Contraceptive	CBD Price	Pharmacy Price
1 cycle of pills	M 1.00	M 4.50
IUD	M 2 .00	(not available)
Foam	M .50	M 19.00 per can
Condoms	Free	M 1.00 for six

There was still concern among some of the staff that this reimbursement system might not be adequate. Therefore, an annual contest was planned to increase motivation through the award of prize money at a ceremony. Two prizes were to be offered. The first would be awarded to the best team. A separate prize was to be offered to the six best agents. Five criteria were outlined for the best team prize. Three of the criteria -- working relationship as a group, working relationship with the community, and working relationship with the clients -- would be assessed during the monthly supervisory visits. The other two criteria -- amount of sales and number of acceptors -- would be taken from the monthly statistics. Performance for the awards to the six best agents would be assessed from independent site visits by the senior management team and the executive director. During these visits, they would talk with community leaders, agents, and clients. The award system and the criteria were explained to all the distributors.

Three months after the program started, Mrs. Tyler decided it was time to give some attention to the incentive scheme.

That same day at lunch in the FPAM canteen, Mr. Armstrong, the project accountant, had brought up a new problem uncovered during a monthly supervisory visit to Gabazzatown.

"Mrs. Tyler," he said, "We've got a problem. We've told the distributors that the most important thing is to serve their clients, but when the clients can't pay it puts them in a difficult position. If they give the client an advance and it is not repaid, the distributor has to pay for the contraceptives out of her or his own pocket. If they refuse to provide the contraceptives, they lose an active user for the project and the woman runs the risk of becoming pregnant."

Mrs. Tyler couldn't think of a solution right away. However, just as she was about to get up from the table an idea came to her. "I've got it," she said. "What we'll do is instruct the agents to advance up to three monthly cycles when clients can't pay. After that time we'll tell them they must report to Betty or you about the outstanding advances. One of you will then follow up with the client to see if they really can't afford the pills. We don't want to be supplying free cycles to people who are using the money to drink Club Beer in the evenings. But if the client really can't afford to pay, Betty or you can declare them indigent, and the pills can be distributed free of charge after that. This will fix part of the problem for the distributor in the short term. We'll have to change the system during the second phase of the project to provide some incentive for the distributors to supply these clients."

"That's a great idea," Mr. Armstrong said. "I think it will work."

Mrs. Tyler smiled. She was in hurry to get to a meeting. "That's what I'm here for. Occasionally I come up with a good idea!" She stood up, leaving Mr. Armstrong drinking his coffee at the table.

A week later, Mr. Somatta, the team leader from Jeffersonville, and his counterpart in Slipyaw-Bossa, Miss Stewart, got together to plan a motivation session for a large group of potential acceptors at the student hall of the university. Their conversation turned to the topic of the awards.

"This award system really bothers me," said Miss Stewart. "I have no idea how they're going to decide who gets the awards. Do you?"

Mr. Somatta responded, "They called us all to a meeting at the beginning of the summer to tell us about the awards, but I haven't heard much since then. I've never been sure how they will decide on the prizes. Anyway, it seems unfair to me because the communities are so different. I've got an agent assigned to upper Broad Street which is 90 percent Moslem. It's nearly impossible to sell them on the idea of family planning."

"That's true," Miss Stewart agreed. "Three of my agents have a similar problem. Their clients aren't home during the day. They either have to work on weekends or late in the evenings. Don't you think that the award should be given to the distributors that show the most commitment?"

"Sure," Mr. Somatta replied. "But how would you measure that?"

"Well, you could give the award to the agents who log the most miles on foot," she said jokingly.

"Seriously, though, I think the differences between the communities make the incentive system a bit unfair," said Mr. Somatta. "Maybe the project should be reimbursing the distributors for their time. Some of the distributors that are in these difficult areas may quit in a few months."

"Talking about incentive systems, I got stuck last week paying for eight cycles of pills out of my own pocket," said Miss Stewart. "This is happening to me every month. I don't want my clients to drop out and get pregnant, but I can't afford to subsidize them, either."

"You know," Mr. Somatta responded, "when we get talking like this, it helps a bit to remember what Miss Elgazan is always telling us. 'Don't think of sales. That's not the important thing. What matters is convincing people that family planning is important for them. Once you've done this, sales will follow'."

"But the system isn't all that fair either," Miss Stewart said. "When we make referrals for IUDs, injectables, or sterilization, we don't get any remuneration. That's a lot of work for nothing."

A couple of months later Mrs. Tyler called her senior staff together. She had decided that it was time to redesign the incentive scheme for the second phase of the project.

Study Questions

1. What are the problems with the current financial incentive scheme?

2. What data would be helpful to evaluate the success of the financial incentive scheme during the first phase of the project?

3. What recommendations would you make for modifications to be made in designing the second phase incentive system?

B) Case Analysis: The Sales Force

This case explores different ways of compensating CBD agents. To a lesser extent, the case also addresses setting prices for contraceptives. As mentioned in the background discussion for this section on community-based distribution, both of these issues are sensitive. The implications of a particular system need to be carefully considered before implementation in a specific program.

The debate over how to pay agents is an interesting one. In this case, FPAM's program starts with two opposite alternatives supported by the two key agencies. A salary system is proposed by Mrs. Tyler and FPAM, and a straight commission is supported by the donors. The system which FPAM develops seeks to combine these two methods. The twenty momambi monthly salary will help to motivate workers initially, and provide some consistent support. Having the agents keep 50 percent of their sales revenue effectively ties their income to performance, while ensuring that they are offered some compensation for their efforts, particularly initially. A potential problem with the current incentive system is that it does not remunerate agents for referrals for IUDs, injectable contraceptives or sterilizations. This could lead to decreased emphasis on these methods, and an inappropriate choice of method for certain clients.

In reaching a compromise between salary and incentives, Mrs. Tyler again demonstrated her negotiating skills. She was open-minded, and primarily committed to finding a feasible solution. This approach combines positive elements of both systems of financial reward, and also introduces the idea of bonuses.

The bonus system of awards and prizes for individual agents and the best team are designed as a further source of incentives. Though it is difficult to measure, Mrs. Tyler has deliberately made the selection process qualitative, as well as quantitative. This is commendable because it motivates agents to provide quality services, and rewards personal skills and group cooperation. It also will help to minimize some of the differences in performance inherent in the variation between neighborhoods. However, there is a lack of clarity as to how the winners will be selected. This seems to have upset some of the staff.

While the pricing system has attempted to keep contraceptives affordable and sells them below the market price, there is clearly the need for a backup system for people who cannot afford to pay. It is unacceptable for agents to use their own resources to provide contraceptives to clients who cannot pay. However, even a short-term lack of cash can have serious consequences for the client and the program.

There is probably little disagreement on what the policy should be. However, implementing a practical solution is more difficult. A temporary solution identified in the case is to have a supervisor certify that a client is indigent. This system has several drawbacks. It requires verification and follow-up from the supervisor. This could potentially require a significant amount of time and effort from people who are already very busy with other responsibilities. Furthermore, establishing a means test which is fair, equitable, and reliable is difficult. Clients certified as "indigent" may resist being labelled in this way, and hesitate to become involved with the program. It should also be noted that casual supervision of the certification process could lead to an opportunity for embezzlement by the agents.

86/Part VI   Financial Control

PART VI   FINANCIAL CONTROL

Overview

Every program needs a financial management system in order to be able to account for the money it receives and spends. The foundation of financial management is the accounting system.

The accounting system presents the financial results of a program's operations over a period of time. A financial statement summarizes the revenues earned and the expenses incurred by the program and ensures that all the money spent by the organization or program is recorded and accounted for. The broad objectives of any accounting system are:

- to ensure that transactions are carried out in accordance with authorized procedures;

- to ensure that transactions are recorded properly in order to maintain accountability for assets and liabilities, and to permit the preparation of financial statements;

- to ensure that access to assets is permitted only in accordance with the management's authorization;

- to ensure that assets are physically verified at regular intervals and that appropriate action is taken in the event of differences.

Setting up an Accounting System and Controlling the Receipt of Money

The first step in setting up an accounting system is to determine how financial transactions will be recorded. To do this, you must design the management procedures that determine how money will flow through the system and how each person who is authorized to handle money will record each financial transaction.

For example, in a community-based distribution program, the CBD agent would record each contraceptive sale on a numbered duplicate receipt. Every month the team leader would collect the money and receipts from the CBD agents. These receipts serve as a record of contraceptive sales; the money collected by the team leader should equal the total amount on the receipts. The team leader would then issue the CBD agent a receipt. This receipt is both proof that the agent has turned over the money she or he has collected and a record that the team leader has received this money. The team leader would then record the amount of money received and contraceptives issued from all the agents. When the team leader turned the money over to the financial manager, the financial manager would issue a receipt for this money. The financial manager would then total the amounts from all team leaders and deposit the money in the bank, recording clearly the source, date, and amount of the money deposited. There is good financial control in this scenario because the flow of money can be traced all the way back to original sale and receipt of money.

Projecting and monitoring expenses and revenues

Another key component for financial management control is the ability to project and monitor expenses and revenues. Projecting and monitoring expenses and revenues is an activity shared by the financial and program managers. The program managers develop a budget and project the revenues during the planning process and the financial managers keep a record of expenses incurred and revenues generated as the program is carried out.

Budgets are detailed projections of the cost of program activities. The budget is usually developed during the planning process. Good planning systems link this budget development with the financial management system. This is important because it is essential for an organization to be able to know exactly how much money it has available to carry out its activities at any given time. The link between the budget developed during the planning process and the financial management system is the chart of accounts. The chart of accounts lists the categories and line items by which revenues and expenses will be recorded. It is best when financial managers and planners work together to develop budget projections because the costs projected during the budget process can be put into a format which is most compatible with the chart of accounts. At the beginning of the year financial managers can set up a system to monitor expenses for each line item against the budgeted projections. In this way both the financial manager and the program manager know how much money they have spent and how much remains.

Estimates of revenues that will be generated through the sale of contraceptives are made during the planning process. These revenues can be allocated to cover all or some of program costs. It is important to keep track of actual revenues and compare them with revenue projections because if actual revenues are less than estimated, managers will need to readjust the level of program activity.

Using Financial Information

Cost and revenue information can be used by managers at many different levels to assess program performance and examine the results of any changes in program procedures, structure or design. The system can provide such information as the cost of resources used, the cost of providing each type of service to clients, or the amount of money generated for different types of services.

With this information, the financial management system can generate management reports that help managers make program adjustments to improve cost-effectiveness and program efficiency.

The next case study, Keeping an Eye on the Money, describes how the financial manager at FPAM set up a financial control system that permitted him to keep track of revenues and expenses and monitor expenses against budget.

CASE 9   KEEPING AN EYE ON THE MONEY

(The following case is divided into three parts.)

Case Learning Points

- Understand how to analyze a financial control system.

- Understand how to develop reporting procedures for all organizational levels.

- Appreciate the difficulties in implementing a system of strict financial controls.

A) Case Study: Keeping an Eye on the Money (I)

In the early days of the CBD project, when it had just received final approval from Pathways and money was made available for project start-up activities, the FPAM Board and Mrs. Tyler interviewed many candidates for the position of Financial Officer of the CBD project. The selection process was long and arduous, and, finally the new financial officer, Mr. Armstrong, reported to work.

Mr. Armstrong was young but extremely well-prepared for his job as the CBD financial officer. He was a graduate of the University of Momonboro and had received postgraduate training in finance in Scotland. Prior to joining the FPAM staff, he had been the financial manager of the Momonboro Consolidated Fish Company. On his first day of work at FPAM, he met with the Executive Director for a short introductory meeting. After welcoming him to the organization and introducing him to the rest of the staff, Mrs. Tyler sat him down on the large couch in her office.

"Mr. Armstrong, I can't tell you how glad I am to have you on board. We have been needing a financial officer for some time and we're way behind schedule. We've got a quarterly report due at the end of the month and we don't even have financial management system in place." Mrs. Tyler readjusted her position on the couch and ignored the telephone ringing on her desk. "The first thing you've got to do after you've read all the project documents is to come up with a financial management system. And it has to be ready by the third week of this month."

Mr. Armstrong nodded, but remained silent.

"I know it sounds like a lot of work, but I really need this now."

The phone rang again and Mrs. Tyler moved from the couch to answer it. She motioned to Mr. Armstrong that she was finished. As he left her office he realized that he wouldn't be able to work his way gradually into his new job.

Back in his office, Mr. Armstrong readjusted his tie. Despite the heat he had always worked in a tie and a starched shirt. He pulled out the project documents and began to read. By the end of his first day, he had set his principal objectives for the system on paper. They were:

- to monitor contraceptive sales by distributors;

- to monitor financial transactions between distributors and team leaders;

- to monitor contraceptive inventory (individual pill types and other products);

- to report on expenditures and on the current balance for each project line item;

- to provide financial data for quarterly Pathways reports.

By the end of the first week, he had the rough outlines of a financial management system drafted on paper.

First, he had written down how he thought the money would be handled in the system.

1. Agents would sell contraceptives, collecting money which they would keep until the team leader's monthly supervisory visit.

2. The team leader would take the money to the monthly supervisory meeting and turn it over to the financial officer.

3. After checking the amounts on the spot, the financial officer would return half of the money collected from the sales to the agents as their commission.

4. The financial officer would deposit the remainder of the money in the FPAM bank account.

For the inventory he wrote:

1. Agents would be issued a certain amount of contraceptives to start with, and black bags to carry their stock.

2. Agents would sell pills, condoms and contraceptive foam to clients.

3. Agents would be restocked either at the monthly supervisory meeting or by a part-time stockperson who would be available to call on distributors at their homes.

Mr. Armstrong then decided to design a system that would account for and monitor these transactions at all levels. Pills were being sold for M 4.50 in the pharmacies and he worried that agents might try to get more money by selling them for more than the one momambi price that FPAM had set. With this potential for abuse, he knew that strict monitoring of financial transactions was necessary.

Study Questions

1. If you were Mr. Armstrong, how would you go about designing a financial management system that meets each of your objectives?

2. How would you prevent agents from overcharging? What receipts would you require?

3. How would you know that the amount of money you received from the team agents was correct?

B) Case Analysis: Keeping an Eye on the Money (I)

In this case, Mr. Armstrong has been given the assignment of design-ing a financial management system from scratch. To make matters more difficult, he has to do it very rapidly in order to put out a quar-terly report, and he must design it in such a way that it will collect the information necessary for this report.

As he designs the system, Mr. Armstrong has to keep several consid-erations in mind. First, he must make sure that he can track all finan-cial transactions and provide financial information to the people who need it. In addition, he has to keep the system simple and workable, so that everyone understands what they are supposed to do, can do it correctly, and can carry out these tasks within a reasonable amount of time. Mr. Armstrong also has to account for the fact that abuses of the system might occur, and to incorporate safeguards against them.

The first thing Mr. Armstrong does is to set objectives for what the system he is designing ought to do. Once he has determined that the system should monitor sales, the financial transactions between agents and team leaders, and the inventory of contraceptives, and provide financial information on expenditures and the current balance, he decides how the money from sales should change hands. It will flow from the agents to the team leaders during the monthly supervisory visits, and to himself at the time of the supervisory meetings, at which time half of the money from each sale will be returned to the agents.

Having decided how the money will flow through the system, Mr. Armstrong decides how the agents will receive and replenish their contraceptive supplies. Now he has to design a simple and workable way to record both the financial and contraceptive inventory trans-actions, get the records of these transactions to the people who need them in a timely fashion, and prevent any financial abuse of the system.

A) Case Study: Keeping an Eye on the Money (II)

Working from his initial outline, Mr. Armstrong designed the following system to track each financial transaction in the CBD program.

1. Agents would be issued a numbered receipt book with numbered duplicate receipts in which to record all sales (see Exhibit 1). For each transaction, one copy of the receipt would be given to the client and the other would be retained by the agent in a numbered book.

2. Team leaders would have similar books in which they would record the money received from their agents. Receipts would be issued to each agent for the total amount of money received. A duplicate copy would be retained in the team leaders' own books and then turned over to the finance officer along with the agents' original receipts at the monthly supervisory meeting.

3. At supervisory meetings, the financial officer would review each agent's records, checking them for accuracy against the team leader's record, before reimbursing the agent for half the value of her or his sales. The financial officer would then ask the agent to sign for receipt of the money.

In order to keep track of inventory, Mr. Armstrong decided to have agents write the specific name of the contraceptive on the receipt. He also devised a simple stock control form for the agents to fill out each month (Exhibit 2). In this way he could check inventory against sales.

4. After returning to FPAM, the financial officer would transfer the individual receipts from each agent to a spreadsheet (Exhibit 3). In this way he would have a record of the total sales of each individual agent, which included the client's name and the amount of money for each type of contraceptive purchased. This system was attractive to Mr. Armstrong because he would be able to spot check individual clients to verify whether the agent had sold contraceptives and at the correct price. (When he worked for the Momonboro Consolidated Fish Co., this type of spreadsheet had proved a valuable tool for adjusting inventories and prices according to sales trends.)

5. Next he prepared a cumulative statement showing contraceptive revenues for each community in the project for each three-month period (Exhibit 4).

In order to report on total CBD project expenditures and the current balance for each line item, he devised a new chart of accounts (Exhibit 5). Using his new list, he created a spreadsheet called "Expenditure Control Analysis" which was a cumulative list of the starting balance, the monthly expenses and the remaining account balances for each line item (Exhibit 6). This permitted him to monitor actual expenses against budget projections for each line item on a monthly basis. For example, if the price of petrol were to rise, he could easily note a rise in the monthly expenditure as compared to previous months. The current balance item would provide information on the implications of this price increase for the completion of project activities.

Finally, using the financial management system he had developed, he was easily able to satisfy the donor agencies requirements for a quarterly financial report.

Study Questions

1. How does this compare with the system you developed?

2. Do you see any potential problems with this system?

3. How has Mr. Armstrong prevented the agents from charging extra for the contraceptives and pocketing the difference?

Exhibit I

FAMILY PLANNING ASSOCIATION
OF MOMONBORO

P.O. BOX 389
PLACATTE, MOMONBORO

Community-Based Distribution

Receipt No. 001837

Date: October 3

Location: Royalton

Received from: Lucy Tuquois

Amount: ₦ 1:00 (in words): One Momambi

Type of Service: Oral Contraceptives Sale

For: .... Quantity: ....

Patricia Tah

Authorized Signature

Exhibit 2

FPAM/CBD Contraceptive Stock Control Form

Name: Patricia Tal   Area: Westport
Zone: Λ   Month: September

Brand Type	Starting Quantity	Quantity Received	Total Stock	Quantity Issue	Balance Quantity on Hand
FEMENAL	85	—	85	4	81
LO-FEMENAL	38	60 LO-FEMENAL	93	7	86
OVRAL	48	—	48	2	46
MICRO-	45	—	45	6	39
CONCEPTROL	3	—	3	3	—
VAG. CREAM	6	—	6	—	6

Financial Intake

Total Pills Sold	19	at	M1.00	each = M	19.00
Total Foam Tabs Sold	3	at	M0.50	each = M	1.50
Total IUDs Sold		at		each = M	
Total Injections Sold		at		each = M	

Exhibit 3

FPAM/CBD Sales Analysis

Area: _Westport_

Date: _September_

Agent/Client Name	Receipt #	Cash	Micro	Foam	L/Foam	F/Tab	F/Cream	
Zelda Brapleh								
Mitete Clark	10034	1.00		1.00				
Anita Basaca	10035	1.00			1.00			
Sitete Paye	10036	1.00		1.00				
Martha Sherman	10037	1.00			1.00			
Yaran Say	10038	2.00			2.00			
Narite Matore	10039	1.00		1.00				
Mary Tugla	10040	1.00	1.00					
Noah Victor	10041	1.00		1.00				
Annie Noah	10042	1.00	1.00					
Marie Dumanis	10043	1.00			1.00			
		11.00	2.00	4.00	5.00			
Patricia Tah								
Annie Brown	1408	1.00		1.00				
Mary Andrew	1409	1.00			1.00			
Lucy Tuquois	1410	1.00	1.00					
Sarah Sisk	1411	1.00		1.00				
Cecilia Lamb	1412	1.00	1.00					
Batusca Toe	1413	1.00		1.00				
Annie Anthony	1414	1.00			1.00			
Alma Targuis	1415	1.00	1.00					
Lopkins Tinto	1416	1.00	1.00					
Linda Duch	1417	1.00			1.00			
Jennie Leah	1418	1.00			1.00			
Mary Kemach	1419	1.00		1.00				
Grace Topay	1420	1.00	1.00					
Mannie Sisk	1421	1.00			1.00			
Benda Wilson	1422	1.00		1.00				
Nancy Johnsen	1423	1.00	1.00					
Mabel Keits	1424	1.00			1.00			
Esther Kin	1425	1.00	1.00					
Susanna Toe	1426	1.50				1.50		
Harriet Leah	1427	1.00			1.00			
		20.50	7.00	5.00	7.00	1.50		

Exhibit 4

CUMULATIVE STATEMENT OF CONTRACEPTIVE
REVENUES FOR EACH COMMUNITY

Monthly Sales Report

Greater Placatte	July	August	Sept	Total	50% of Total
Bossa Community	M 84.00	M 59.00	M 71.00	M 214.00	M 107.00
East Middleton	138.50	241.00	166.00	545.50	272.75
Clearwater Comm.	147.50	123.00	130.50	400.50	200.25
Slipyaw	47.00	57.50	45.50	150.00	75.00
Royalton	157.00	125.50	120.50	406.00	203.00
Newkrutown	402.50	188.00	177.50	778.00	389.00
St. Johnsville	405.50	257.50	258.00	916.00	458.00
Gabazzatown	447.00	240.00	218.50	905.50	457.75
Total	1838.50	1319.50	1187.50	4345.00	2172.75
50 percent	919.25	659.75	593.75	2172.75	
East Middleton Clinic			31.00	31.00	15.50
Newkrutown			50.50	50.50	25.25
Ely Clinic			6.00	6.00	3.00
Total					43.75
Grand Total					M 2216.50

Exhibit 5

FAMILY PLANNING ASSOCIATION OF MOMONBORO
COMMUNITY-BASED DISTRIBUTON PROJECT
Chart of Accounts

Code Description

ASSETS

110	Cash on Hand
111	Bank Account -- Tradevco
112	Petty Cash

RECEIVABLES

115	International Assistance for Child Spacing
116	Staff-debtors
117	Customers
118	Other Grants
119	Pathways Grant Control

INVENTORY

125	Contraceptives
126	Drugs and Medical Supplies
127	Stationery and Supplies

FIXED ASSETS

135	Office Equipment -- Typewriter
136-1	Furniture and Fixture -- Cabinet
136-2	Furniture and Fixture -- Chairs
136-3	Furniture and Fixture -- Desks
137-1	Clinic Equip. -- Exam Couch
137-2	Clinic Equip. -- Anglepoise Lamps
137-3	Clinic Equip. -- Blood Pressure Apparatus
137-4	Clinic Equip. -- Thermometer
137-5	Clinic Equip. -- Weighing Scales

LIABILITIES

150	Accounts Payable
151	IACS/FPAM
152	Withholdings -- Income Tax
153	Withholdings -- National Reconst. Tax
154	Withholdings -- Health Tax
155	Withholdings -- Development Tax

INCOME (REVENUE)

170	Pathways Grant
171	Contraceptive Sales
171-1	Greater Placatte
171-2	Newkrutown
171-3	East Middleton
171-4	Clearwater

Code Description

171-5	Royalton
171-6	Bossa
171-7	Slipyaw
171-8	St. Johnsville
171-9	Gabazzatown

OTHER INCOME

180	Registration Fees
182-2	Laboratory Fees
182-3	Clinical Fees
183	Membership Dues
184	Donations
185	Discount Received

EQUITY

190	Capital Investment (Grant)
191	Retained Earnings

EXPENSES

300	Program Officer's Salary
301	Accountant's Salary

BENEFITS

303-1	Program Officer's Contract Allowance
303-2	Accountant's Contract Allowance
304-1	Program Officer's Social Security
304-2	Accountant's Social Security
305-1	Program Officer's Medical Insurance
305-2	Accountant's Medical Insurance

FEES AND HONORARIA

307	Accounting Technical Support Assistance
308	Evaluation Consultancy
309	Team Best Performance Prize Award
310	CBD Best Performance Prize Award

GENERAL ADMINISTRATION

312	Postage, Telephone, Telex, Telegram
313	Accounting Books
314	Bank Charges
315	Stationery and Supplies
316	Claim, Port, Handling Charges

Code Description

TRAVEL AND ASSOCIATED EXPENSES
318 Fuel and Travel -- Central Program Staff
319 Fuel and Travel -- Program Director
320 Fuel and Travel -- Program Coordinator
321 Fuel and Travel -- Team Leaders
322 Fuel and Travel -- Distributors

SUPPLIES AND EQUIPMENT
324-1 CBD -- Badges
324-2 CBD -- Bags
325 Expendable Clinic Supplies
326 Rain Boots and Coats

PURCHASED SERVICES
330 Printing Record Keeping Forms

EDUCATION AND TRAINING

SEMINAR -- CBD COMMITTEE MEMBERS
331 Lunch Allowance
332 Training Materials
333 Transportation Allowance

TRAINER'S WORKSHOP
334 Lunch Allowance
335 Training Materials

CBD -- WORKERS AND TRAINERS
336 Lunch Allowance
337 Training Materials
337-1 Graduation Ceremonies (Refreshments)

TEAM LEADERS TRAINING
338 Lunch and Transportation Allowance
339 Training Materials

DISTRIBUTORS AND TRAINERS COURSE
340 Lunch and Transportation Allowance
341 Training Materials

Code Description

DEVELOPMENT OF IE&C MATERIALS
342-1 Printing Material, Brochures
343 Posters for Literate and Non-Literate Audience
344 Radio Spots, Public Services

REFERRAL AND BACK-UP CLINIC STAFF TRAINING
345 Lunch and Transport Allowance
346 Lunch for Facilitators
347 Training Materials

OTHER EXPENSES
348 Tuition Fees (Study or Seminar Tour)
349 Air Ticket (Flight Fare)
350 Per Diem (Foreign)
351 Sundry or Related Expenses
352 Local Air Fare
353 Per Diem (Local)
354 Rental Fees

CODES SUMMARY
110 - 140 .... Assets
150 - 160 .... Liabilities
170 - 180 .... Income
190 - 200 .... Equity
300 - 400 .... Expenses

Exhibit 6

Community–Based Distribution Project

Expenditures Control Analysis

(Only the first page is shown)

Salaries/Wages	May–July Prev. Balance*	August Expenditures	September Expenditures	October Expenditures	Total Expenditures	Current Balance
Program Officer -- CBD	7,440.—	800.—	800.—	800.—	2,400.—	5,040.—
Junior Accountant -- CBD	9,040.—	800.—	800.—	800.—	2,400.—	6,640.—
	16,480.—	1,600.—	1,600.—	1,600.—	4,800.—	11,680.—
Benefits						
Contract Allowance	1,648.—	160.—	240.—	80.—	480.—	1,168.—
National Job Security	512.—					512.—
Medical Insurance	840.—	142.50		142.50	285.—	555.—
	3,000.—	302.50	240.—	222.50	765.—	2,235.—
Fees/Honoraria						
Training Support	2,000.—					2,000.—
Evaluation Consultant	300.—					300.—
Annual Team Awards	1,750.—					1,750.—
Best CBD Awards	1,500.—					1,500.—
	5,550.—					5,550.—
General Admin. & Services						
Postage and Telephone	1,527.92	136.95	8.55	46.—	191.50	1,336.42
Accounting Books	514.75	243.—			243.—	71.75
Bank Charges	570.—		1.60		1.60	568.40
Stationery and Supplies	372.75	18.50	10.—	58.75	87.25	285.50
Claims & Handling Charges	648.83	.80			.80	648.03
	3,434.25	399.25	20.15	104.75	524.15	2,910.10
Project Staff Expenses						
Food and Transportation	7,200.—		1,010.—	465.—	1,475.—	5,725.—
Project Director	400.—		200.—			200.—
Project Coordinator	960.—		160.—		160.—	800.—
Team Leader	5,760.—	132.10	414.35	248.65	795.10	4,964.90
Distributors	11,520.—	1,067.30	2,120.—	1,060.—	4,247.30	7,272.70
	25,840.—	1,199.40	3,904.35	1,773.65	6,877.40	18,962.60
Supplies and Equipment						
Typewriter	70.52					70.52
Desks	75.93					75.93
Chairs	53.60					53.60
Filing Cabinet	62.03					62.03
Raincoats and Boots	1,430.—					1,430.—
CBD Badges	110.—					110.—
CBD Bags	300.—					300.—
Angle Lamps	210.—					210.—
Blood Pressure Apparatus	80.—					80.—
Thermometers	100.—					100.—
Weighing Scales	199.50					199.50
Expendable Clinic Supplies	4,200.—		1,844.50	599.55	2,444.35	1,755.65
	6,891.58		1,844.50	599.55	2,444.35	4,447.23

* Previous Balance = Projected expenses for year minus cumulative expenses to date

B) Case Analysis: Keeping an Eye on the Money (II)

In this section, we see in detail the system which Mr. Armstrong has set up. Has he addressed all the objectives and concerns he set out before he began?

There seems to be a clear flow of information from the individual agents to the financial officer, who assembles and analyzes the information for reports. The system is not all that simple, and the agents have to wait until the next monthly supervisory meeting before they can get their 50 percent commission. But the system ought to prevent abuses because both the client and the team leader will receive copies of each sales receipt, so the agent cannot charge the client extra, and because the receipts are numbered, it will be evident if one is missing. Any discrepancy would show up on the spread sheet.

One of Mr. Armstrong's objectives for the system is to monitor sales. Each sale is recorded on a receipt, which is reviewed during the monthly visit by the team leader who records the total amount of money collected on a receipt. A copy of this receipt goes to the finance officer. All of this information is then transferred to the financial officer's spreadsheet. This series of receipts lets Mr. Armstrong monitor the financial transactions between the distributors and the team leaders (objective 2) as well as the contraceptive sales (objective 1).

In order to monitor contraceptive inventory (objective 3), the distributors are asked to write the specific name of the contraceptive on the receipt. To find out about expenditures and the current balance for each project line item (objective 4), Mr. Armstrong would refer to the Expenditure Control Analysis spread sheet. Finally, the financial data necessary for the quarterly Pathways reports (objective 5) would be drawn from the cumulative statement of contraceptive revenues for each community in the project for each three-month period.

A) Case Study: Keeping an Eye on the Money (III)

Two months later things were working well, but Mr. Armstrong had a nose for sniffing out problems and setting things straight. For one thing, he found that he was spending a tremendous amount of time handling money. He decided to delegate financial control of the agents to the team leader. During the third month, he changed the system so that the team leader collected only 50 percent of the agents' sales. This innovation meant that Mr. Armstrong could reduce his direct supervision of agents. Now he could simply check the team leaders' summary sheet during the monthly supervisory meeting without compromising financial control.

He had also noted that on the agents' receipts, TYPE OF SERVICE was often being filled out as "pills" rather than the specific brand and type (Lo-Ovral, Ovral, etc.). This presented an inventory control problem because he needed to keep track of sales by product type. He brought this to the agents' attention and tried to improve compliance. Eventually, however, he gave up trying to change the agents' habits and decided that during the second phase of the project he would redesign the receipt so that the agents could check off the type of pill dispensed.

There was a third and more serious problem which became clearer as the project became more successful. The spreadsheet which Mr. Armstrong had developed from his experience at the fish company was becoming a heavy burden. It took an enormous amount of time to prepare, and was giving him some details that he didn't need and some that he could find elsewhere. He knew that he had good inventory control through his stock control form and that he could get names for periodic spot checks of clients from the agents' receipts. Therefore, he felt increasingly comfortable with the idea of consolidating the spreadsheet, omitting the individual clients' names, and just tracking total sales and inventory for each agent.

B) Case Analysis: Keeping an Eye on the Money (III)

Mr. Armstrong has found that the financial management system he devised is more complex than it needs to be, so he has made some adjustments to make it more efficient. He has found that he does not have to have all the money from sales turned over to him; the team leaders can just collect half. This approach probably has the added benefit of pleasing the distributors, who will thus receive their commission for each sale immediately. In making this change, Mr. Armstrong does not lose any control over the system; the system of receipts remains in place, and he receives the same information.

Mr. Armstrong has shown an important characteristic of good management: flexibility. He needs information on what brand of contraceptive is being sold in order to maintain an accurate inventory, but although he asked the distributors several times to write the brand on the receipt, it was rarely done. Rather than continuing to insist with little result, Mr. Armstrong has taken another approach, one that is appropriate to the situation and has a greater chance of success. The new coupon books will have all the brands listed and the distributors will just have to check one off.

He was equally sensible and flexible about his spreadsheet. Although it had worked well at the Momonboro Consolidated Fish Company and it had seemed like a good idea for the CBD project, Mr. Armstrong soon realized that it took far too much time to fill out and provided him with information he didn't need. Again, he was not resistant to change, kept a clear view of the situation, and eliminated unnecessary steps.

All of Mr. Armstrong's modifications have brought him closer to one of his original concerns: that the system should be simple and workable.

PART VII   COMMUNITY-BASED DISTRIBUTION
START-UP KIT

This is a condensed version of the information presented in the main text of this book. This section is intended for easy reference as you start up your own CBD program, so that you can quickly see all the steps involved in setting up such a program.

At the beginning of each of the six sections of this start-up kit is a checklist of all the steps which need to be completed and which are explained in that section. Each section gives the page numbers where a complete explanation can be found.

There is a complete checklist at the end of the start-up kit starting on page 137.

— **Momonboro** —

You will find examples from the Momonboro program in the boxes like this one.

I. PLANNING   DONE

STRATEGIC PLANNING

MISSION of the organization

GOALS of the organization

WHERE, WHAT and HOW of the organization

OPERATIONAL PLANNING

STRATEGIES, OBJECTIVES, and TARGETS for each goal

ENVIRONMENTAL ANALYSIS

Identify:

INTERNAL FACTORS affecting the new program

EXTERNAL FACTORS affecting the new program

OBSTACLES (Internal and External)

OPPORTUNITIES (Internal and External)

Divide Obstacles into:

Those which can be OVERCOME

Those which can be REDUCED

Those we must work AROUND

Identify PROBLEMS which could occur and proposed SOLUTIONS

Develop a LIST OF PEOPLE who can influence the program's success

Meet with the people on this LIST

Get the support of COMMUNITY LEADERS

STRATEGIC PLANNING (page 10) is the process organizations use to decide on the basic purpose of the organization (the mission) and the organization's long-term goals. Strategic planning is important for developing a thorough understanding of how the CBD program will contribute to the organization's mission and goals, and what the future impact of a CBD program will be on the organization.

I.   What is the **MISSION** of the organization?

—————————————————————————————— **Momonboro** —

MISSION: To deliver family planning services to women of reproductive age.

II. What are the organization's **GOALS**?

—————————————————————————————— **Momonboro** —

GOALS:
1. To increase the number of couples using modern methods of contraception.

2. To improve the accessibility of family planning services to rural and urban couples.

3. To educate and assist more couples to space their births by two years.

III. **WHERE** is the organization now?

WHERE does the organization want to be in five to ten years?

WHAT is the organization trying to achieve?

HOW can the organization get there?

Momonboro

WHERE the organization is: FPAM is now twenty years old. 5.6 percent of eligible women are using modern contraceptive methods. Family planning services are still inaccessible to many.

WHERE it should be in five years: The delivery of high quality family planning services should be expanded to 25 percent of women of reproductive age in Momonboro.

WHAT the organization is trying to achieve: Making family planning services affordable and accessible so that couples can space their pregnancies to have healthy children, and limit their pregnancies so they have the number of children they want; making the FPAM known to women who know about family planning but don't currently know where to get services.

HOW it will get there: Making services more accessible through community-based distribution and social marketing; increasing public information efforts and advertising.

OPERATIONAL PLANNING (page 11) takes the broad goals which were developed in the strategic planning process and develops the concrete objectives and strategies necessary to achieve these goals.

For each of the organization's **GOALS**, state its:

STRATEGIES: how each goal will be achieved

OBJECTIVES: what results need to be achieved when and by whom in order to meet the goals

TARGETS: exactly what must be done, written in numerical terms

The number of goals, strategies, objectives, and targets you have will vary from what is presented here, but you should be able to use the same basic format.

Momonboro

GOAL 1:   To increase the percentage of women using a modern method of family planning.

STRATEGY 1:   Begin a pilot CBD program in urban areas.

OBJECTIVE 1:   To increase the percentage of women using a modern method of family planning from 5.6 percent to 25 percent in five years in the target areas.

TARGET 1:   Recruit and train approximately sixty CBD agents and six team leaders.

TARGET 2:   Each CBD agent should recruit at least ten new acceptors each month.

TARGET 3:   Family planning acceptor dropout rate should be kept below 30 percent.

ENVIRONMENTAL ANALYSIS (page 12) Before a program can be developed, the planners must understand the environment in which the program will operate and the factors in the environment which may help or hinder the program.

Collect information on the factors within (**INTERNAL**) and outside (**EXTERNAL**) the organization which will have an impact on the proposed new program. Examples of some subject areas you should consider are listed; you will think up others which relate specifically to your situation.

--- **Momonboro** ---

INTERNAL

1. Clinic staff working at capacity.
2. FPAM has branches in nine counties; eventually each branch could have CBD.
3. Field staff can be a useful resource in planning CBD in their areas.
4. FPAM staff are experienced in IEC work.
5. 85 percent of FPAM budget is dependent on International Planned Parenthood Federation. Other sources needed for special projects.
6. Ministry of Health clinics are able to handle new acceptors coming in for initial visit.
7. FPAM Evaluation Officer already overburdened.

EXTERNAL

1. Strengthened relationships with Ministries of Health, Planning, Education, and Information.
2. Population's level of knowledge of family planning and the benefits of childspacing high (72 percent know about a modern method).
3. Women are interested in using modern contraceptives, but few visit clinic due to a) long wait, b) high cost of transportation, c) loss of time from domestic responsibilities, d) long distances between home and clinic.
4. 33 percent of women in union want to space their pregnancies, 17 percent want no more children.
5. Less than half of women know where they can get a contraceptive method; 12 percent are worried about side effects; 12 percent don't know any modern methods.
6. City clinics are not accessible to rural women (75 percent of the population is rural), and accessibility is a problem even in urban areas.
7. Ministry of Health's budget is decreasing due to country's financial crisis.

Which of these are **OBSTACLES** to the new program, and which are **OPPORTUNITIES?** Opportunities are important resources, material or otherwise, which can be used to benefit the program. Obstacles (such as shortages or regulations or social barriers) can cause problems for the new program. Some examples are provided. Again, this is just the basic format; the number of obstacles and opportunities will vary.

Momonboro

INTERNAL

OBSTACLES

1. Clinic staff working at capacity.
2. 85 percent of budget is dependent on International Planned Parenthood Federation, other sources needed for special projects.
3. Evaluation officer already overburdened.

OPPORTUNITIES

1. FPAM has branches in nine counties; eventually each could replicate CBD.
2. Field staff are a useful resource in planning CBD in their areas.
3. Staff are experienced in IEC work.
4. MOH clinics able to handle new acceptors coming for initial visit.

— **Momonboro** —

EXTERNAL

OBSTACLES

1. Women are interested in using modern contraceptives, but few visit clinic due to a) long wait, b) high cost of transportation, c) loss of time from domestic responsibilities, d) long distances between home and clinic.
2. Less than half of women know where they can get a contraceptive method.
3. Less than 20 percent of women have ever used contraceptives, only 8 percent using a method now.
4. 12 percent of women are worried about side effects.
5. 12 percent of women don't know any modern methods.
6. City clinics are not accessible to rural women (75 percent of the population is rural), and accessibility is a problem even in urban areas.
7. Ministry of Health's budget is decreasing due to country's financial crisis.
8. Women reluctant to make contraceptive decisions without consulting husband.

OPPORTUNITIES

1. Strengthened relationships with Ministries of Health, Planning, Education, and Information.
2. Population's level of knowledge of family planning and child spacing benefits very high.
3. 33 percent of women in union want to space their pregnancies, 17 percent want no more children.

Now divide the obstacles into three groups: those which can be **OVERCOME,** those which can be **REDUCED,** and those which you must **WORK AROUND.**

Momonboro

Obstacles which can be OVERCOME

1. Women not using clinic due to: a) long wait, b) high cost of transport, c) loss of time from domestic responsibilities, d) long distance between home and clinic.
2. Less than half of eligible women know where they can get a family planning method.
3. Less than 20 percent of women have ever used contraceptives; only 8 percent using now.
4. Women reluctant to make contraceptive decision without husband.

Solutions

1. a) CBD agent will come to them, only have to go to clinic once, b) CBD agent will come to them, c) CBD agent visits are short after initial visit, d) CBD agent will come to them.
2. Women will get better information through CBD agent visits and advertising.
3. CBD agents will make methods better known and more acceptable.
4. CBD agent will discuss methods with wife and husband together.

Obstacles which can be REDUCED

1. 85 percent of the budget is dependent on International Planned Parenthood Federation, need other sources for special projects.
2. 12 percent of women are worried about contraceptive's side effects.
3. 12 percent of women don't know any method of contraception.
4. Poor accessibility of clinics to city and rural populations.

How to reduce the problem

1. Look for more than one funding agency, so less vulnerable; raise some revenue from contraceptive sales.
2. CBD agents will explain side effects, clinic staff will take care of problems.
3. CBD agents will visit homes to explain methods.
4. CBD agents will reduce the need for clinics (after initial visit for pill).

```
 ─────────────────────────────────────────── Momonboro ─
| Obstacles we must WORK AROUND                          |
|                                                        |
| 1. Clinic staff working at capacity.                   |
| 2. Evaluation officer overburdened.                    |
| 3. Ministry of Health's budget decreasing due to       |
|    country's financial woes.                           |
|                                                        |
| How to work around them                                |
|                                                        |
| 1. There will be some increase of initial visits --    |
|    perhaps can find new volunteers if necessary.        |
| 2. Have agents and team leaders do more self-          |
|    evaluation and data preparation at own level.        |
| 3. CBD agent handle as much on their own as they can   |
|    (i.e. counseling on side effects).                  |
```

While planning the program, try to think of all the **PROBLEMS** which could occur as you develop and implement your program. Think of the ways you would deal with these problems. By making up such a contingency plan, you will be able to deal with problems quickly and efficiently when they arise.

```
 ─────────────────────────────────────────── Momonboro ─
| PROBLEMS which could occur                             |
|                                                        |
| 1. Poor performance of CBD agents.                     |
| 2. Resistance of community leaders.                    |
|                                                        |
| How to deal with them                                  |
|                                                        |
| 1. Find out problem; motivate, train or replace.       |
| 2. Involve them early with questionnaire, meeting and   |
|    asking advice on CBD agents.                        |
```

At all stages of program planning and implementation, it is important to seek the ideas, advice and sometimes blessing of the **PEOPLE WHO CAN INFLUENCE THE PROGRAM'S SUCCESS**. These people could be in various government ministries, in funding agencies, in similar family planning programs, the staff of your program or organization, influential members of the community (including local leaders, religious leaders and health and family planning workers), and those which the program will serve. Make a list of all these influential people, and be sure to contact them. And don't forget to get the **SUPPORT OF COMMUNITY LEADERS**.

Momonboro

PEOPLE WHO CAN INFLUENCE
THE CBD PROGRAM'S SUCCESS

CONTACTED
FOR ADVICE

1. Sam Ford ✓

2. Heads of the MOH clinics who will receive referrals from CBD program. ✓

3. Professor Pedipaw ✓

4. Community leaders ✓

5. Religious leaders ✓

6. Mayors and other political leaders ✓

7. Officials of the MOH ✓

8. FPAM staff ✓

II. DEVELOPING THE PROGRAM

DONE

Involve your STAFF

Conduct NEEDS ASSESSMENT of the community

Select CBD AGENTS

Train CBD AGENTS

Set up RESUPPLY SYSTEM

Choose CONTRACEPTIVE METHODS to distribute

Be sure to **INVOLVE YOUR STAFF** in the planning process, from the initial conceptualization through all of its stages. For example, discuss intial strategies and plans at staff meetings, circulate project status updates to the staff, provide opportunities for staff members to meet with community leaders, and provide examples of similar programs conducted by other organizations.

— **Momonboro** —

When she was planning the CBD program, Mrs. Tyler sought the advise of her staff as to whether sending out a survey was the best way to initiate contact with the comunities, and what communities to select for the program. The staff worked with the visiting experts to plan the project, and were involved in the writing of the proposal.

You should conduct a **NEEDS ASSESSMENT** (p. 28) of the area in which you plan to have your CBD program. Some information may already exist in the form of demographic surveys. You may need to conduct a small local survey. Your needs assessment should determine:

- the community's demographic structure;

- the community's family planning needs;

- current usage of contraception;

- awareness of and demand for contraceptives;

- community perception of contraception;

- the level of interest in such a program;

- existing family planning services;

- the administrative and political structure of the community;

- how the program should be introduced to increase its chances for success;

- whether that community should be selected for the program.

--- **Momonboro** ---

NEEDS ASSESSMENT: Little information is available on the region in which the CBD program will take place, so the planners have to use the nationwide information which is available.

- Unmet demand exists for family planning services (17 percent want no more children, 33 percent want to space births, 72 percent know about modern methods, only 7 percent using them).

- Some services are provided by MOH clinics (FP staff there trained by FPAM); need to coordinate about new acceptors initial appointments.

- Population is 15 percent Christian, 15 percent Muslim, remainder traditional religion.

- Community perception of family planning is largely favorable.

- Existing family planning services within MOH clinics not used to capacity.

Community perception of your CBD program and its legitimacy will determine whether the program is successful or not. The community's opinion may be heavily dependent on how they view the CBD agents, so **SELECTION OF DISTRIBUTORS** is critically important. Distributors should be known and respected in the community. Talk to your influential people and find out what characteristics they would like to see in a CBD agent before you begin the selection and hiring process. For example, in some areas a married woman might be the most effective agent; in others, a young woman or a male/female team might get the best results.

--- **Momonboro** ---

SELECTION CRITERIA FOR CBD AGENTS

1. Mature and respected resident of the community.
2. Must have an interest in family planning, as demonstrated by previous or present practice of a contraceptive method.
3. Must be able to speak at least one local language.
4. Must have completed 7th grade.

The CBD agents will need **TRAINING**. At a minimum, they should receive training and practice in:

- basic physiology;
- how the methods which they will be distributing work;
- effective ways to approach and communicate with people in the community;
- how to operate resupply and record-keeping systems.

They should also know:

- how the whole CBD program will work;
- how to use checklists to assess the safety of methods for clients;
- when to refer a client to a professional health provider.

Community trust in the program will, in part, be dependent on the CBD agents always having supplies of the contraceptive methods which their clients want. **RESUPPLY SYSTEMS** are thus a very important part of the program.

In planning your program, make sure that:

- you have a reliable and operational resupply system, especially in remote rural areas;

- the resupply system is closely linked with the systems of record-keeping and supervision.

Address the following questions as you plan the resupply system:

- How will the CBD agents know when they receive their resupply how many cycles of pills etc. they will need for the period until the next resupply?

- What do the CBD agents do if they run out of contraceptive supplies? Borrow from another agent?

- Should agents always have a reserve supply? How much would be in that reserve?

Momonboro

RESUPPLY SYSTEM: The CBD agents in Momonboro receive new contraceptive supplies from FPAM at their monthly supervisory meetings.

In many countries, the **TYPES OF CONTRACEPTIVE METHODS** which CBD workers can provide are decided by policies set by the Ministry of Health or other government organizations. In most CBD programs, distributors supply condoms, foams and resupplies of oral contraceptives, and refer clients to a clinic for IUDs, injectables, implants, and sterilization. With additional training, CBD agents could provide oral contraceptives without a clinic visit, and injections.

Momonboro

TYPES OF CONTRACEPTIVE METHODS: The CBD program in Momonboro distributes oral contraceptives, contraceptive foam, and condoms, and refers clients to a clinic for IUDs, injectable contraceptives and sterilizations.

III.   DESIGNING THE MANAGEMENT INFORMATION SYSTEM

DONE

Identify INFORMATION USERS at every level

Identify INFORMATION needed at every level

Identify HOW MANAGERS WILL USE THE INFORMATION

    Evaluation of CBD agents and of the program

    Indicators of Program Performance

Design DATA COLLECTION FORMS

Design REPORTING FORMATS for all levels

Train AGENTS, TEAM LEADERS, AND SUPERVISORS to collect, report and analyze information at their level

A **MANAGEMENT INFORMATION SYSTEM** (p. 37) provides the data and feedback which permit organizations to operate effectively. This information is essential for:

- monitoring;
- evaluation;
- regulating the performance of individual staff members;
- inventory and resupply;
- information for external use (contraceptive prevalence rates, program performance, etc.).

Designing a management information system is a long and detailed process. You want to collect all the necessary information, but not extra information that you don't really need. In designing the system, remember to:

- involve all the people who will use the information for decision making;

- involve all the people who will gather and process the data;

- allow the system to incorporate the various interrelated functions of the organization, such as financial control, evaluation, resupply, staff monitoring and supervision, and reporting;

- make the system flexible enough to allow for modifications as the needs of the program and the users evolve;

- keep the information as brief and concise as possible;

- make sure that the information is also used at the level at which it is collected.

IDENTIFY THE INFORMATION USERS

To decide what information needs to be included:

- identify the users of the system at every level;

- look at:

  - what decisions are made in the organization;

  - who makes these decisions;

  - what information these people need to make informed decisions.

--- **Momonboro** ---

Mr. Alphonse, the statistical officer at FPAM, was given the responsibility of helping Mrs. Tyler to prepare the management information system component of the CBD project. Mr. Alphonse studied the project activities and objectives, the organization chart for project staff, and the project staff job descriptions. He identified all the levels in the system and listed all the information which he thought was needed to manage the program effectively at each level.

FPAM staff designed the CBD agent record, the team leader's monthly report form, and the CBD program officer's monthly report form. Later, Mr. Alphonse found he was frustrated by not having direct access to the information which was being collected, and thought the system might work better if he could get the data first and analyze it.

IDENTIFY THE INFORMATION NEEDED AT EVERY LEVEL

In a CBD program, there are at least three levels of responsibility: the CBD agent, the team leader, and the program officer. Each needs different types of information.

The CBD agent should collect information on:

- basic client characteristics (name/address/sex/age);
- type of contraceptive distributed to each client;
- money collected and outstanding bills;
- number of information and education contacts made;
- number of referrals by method;
- number of dropouts and reason for discontinuation.

The team leader or supervisor needs to collect from each CBD agent information on:

- the number of contacts;
- the number of effective referrals;
- the number of dropouts;
- the number of active users;
- monies collected and outstanding.

The CBD program officer will need to know:

- usage of different commodities for resupply;
- performance indicators (listed above);
- comparative data between agents and teams;
- income generated.

The data should be reported both upward to the project director, and downward to the team leaders and agents through monthly feedback to each team on their performance. Information on program performance should also be shared periodically with the community leaders.

Momonboro

In Momonboro, the CBD agents collect information on:
    date of first CBD service
    name and address of client
    client's information
        age
        sex
        level of education
        number of children living
    contraceptives distributed
        pills
            new acceptor
            continuing acceptor
            quantity
        foam/cream/paste I
            new acceptor
            continuing acceptor
            quantity
        foam/cream/paste II
            new acceptor
            continuing acceptor
            quantity
        condoms
            new acceptor
            continuing acceptor
            quantity
    referrals made
        medical check up
            pills
            IUD
            injectable
        sterilization
            female
            male
        side effects
        natural family planning
    number of contacts made
    months (year) and number of referrals

Momonboro

The team leader collects information on:
    name of agent
    zone
    number of contacts
    contraceptives distributed:
        pills
            new acceptors
            continuing acceptors
            quantity
        foam tablets
            new acceptors
            continuing acceptors
            quantity
        condoms
            new acceptors
            continuing acceptors
            quantity
    effective referrals
        pills
        IUD
        injectables
        sterilization
            male
            female
    drop outs
        side effects
        natural family planning

IDENTIFY HOW MANAGERS WILL USE THE INFORMATION

It is essential that the program have an effective **Evaluation** (page 38) component. Program evaluation can occur at a number of levels:

- self-evaluation by CBD agents;

- evaluation of agent performance by supervisors;

- an internal or external evaluation team assessing the program as a whole.

— Momonboro —

The CBD agents are prevented from doing self-evaluation because their data collection forms are hard to read and use.

Indicators (page 39) of program performance can include:

- total number of active family planning acceptors;

- number of client contacts;

- number of new acceptors;

- number of dropouts;

- number of clinic referrals;

- average length of client contraceptive use;

- quantity of sales of different methods.

You can make these program measures into ratios, such as client contacts per new user, in order to judge program effectiveness.

— Momonboro —

The INDICATORS which the CBD program is currently looking at most closely are the number of people contacted, the number of new acceptors, and by the end of the case studies, the ratio of contacts to acceptors and the dropout rate.

The physical **DESIGN OF DATA COLLECTION FORMS** is very important (page 40). Forms must be:

- easy to carry;
- clear;
- uncluttered;
- quick and easy to use;
- when possible, designed so that data only needs to be entered once.

Forms can be made easier to use by color coding and graphics, when resources allow. For non-literate CBD agents, forms using pictures and simple counts can be used. Be sure to field test them with the agents as you develop them. If possible, forms should include information not only on what type of contraceptive clients are using, but also when they will need a resupply.

Momonboro

Despite the involvement of FPAM in developing the data collection forms, the agents themselves find the forms clumsy and difficult to read. The opinions of the data collectors should always be taken into account and acted on whenever possible, because if they find the forms difficult or unusable, the forms will not serve the program as they are intended to.

When you **DESIGN THE REPORTING FORMATS**, make sure not only that they are as clear and easy to use as the data collection forms, but also that they contain information appropriate for the level of the person collecting the information.

Momonboro

In the Momonboro reporting forms, the CBD agent lists the contraceptive information by family planning acceptor. The team leaders don't need to know who all the acceptors are as they don't need to visit them, so their form lists the contraceptive sales information by CBD agent; that way, they can see how well each agent is doing, which is what they need to know. The project director is not interested in each individual CBD agent; she or he needs to see how well things are going in each project area, so on her or his form the contraceptive sales information is listed by area. (See page 99)

The CBD agents, team leaders and supervisors all need to be trained to carry out their responsiblities effectively.

When you **TRAIN CBD AGENTS, TEAM LEADERS, AND SUPERVISORS** to collect, report, and analyze information at their level, make sure they understand how to fill out the forms correctly and know the schedule of when to submit the forms.

Momonboro

The CBD Agents were trained in the following areas during a two-week course:

- the aims and objectives of the CBD project;

- the health, economic and social benefits of family planning;

- basic human reproduction;

- family planning methods;

- side effects, contraindications and complications;

- family planning information and education;

- screening and counselling of potential clients;

- follow-up visits and client referrals;

- distribution of contraceptives using a checklist;

- community and household mapping;

- dealing with rumors about family planning;

- using CBD reporting forms.

The CBD team leaders underwent this training also and received an additional three days of training on community mapping, target setting, supervision, reporting, and basic accounts.

IV.   SUPERVISION

DONE

Build a SUPERVISORY STRUCTURE:

Develop a SUPERVISORY SCHEDULE

Provide regular FEEDBACK

Set TARGETS for CBD agents

It is important to **BUILD A FORMAL SYSTEM OF SUPERVISION (page 66)** into a program, that is, who supervises whom and how. The structure of a supervisory system for a program is determined by:

- the background of the person being supervised;
- the complexity of the task;
- the personal style of both the supervisor and the worker;
- the atmosphere of the organization;
- the culture in which the program is operating.

Supervision is especially important in CBD programs, as the agents may have limited training and experience in the technical aspects of their work, in working effectively in a community, and in reporting accounting procedures. Supervisory visits can be used to provide clarification and on-going instruction in technical, outreach, and reporting functions, as well as solving problems and motivating the agents. Because of the distances between agents, supervision is often conducted in groups, which means that the agents can share their experiences and learn from one another.

The CBD supervisor will need a **SUPERVISORY SCHEDULE** which lists who is to be visited when and what the meeting will be about. How often supervisory visits need to be made will vary according to the availability of transportation and the distances involved, how long the program has been in operation, and what tasks are performed by the supervisor on the visit. It is important to schedule visits in advance. A general rule is to schedule supervisory visits at least every three months.

Supervision should include **REGULAR FEEDBACK** from the program officer to the team leaders and agents so that they know how well they are doing and how to improve their performance if need be.

Momonboro

The CBD agents are supervised by the team leaders and by the CBD program officer. The CBD team leaders are also supervised by the CBD program officer. The team leaders visit the CBD agents once a month and copy down the necessary information, and the agents and the team leaders have monthly supervisory meetings with the CBD program officer, when problems and concerns are raised and dealt with. Betty Amaya, CBD Program Officer, and Ester Elgazan, Program Officer for Service Delivery, are good at dealing with questions and giving the agents positive feedback. During these supervisory visits, they test the agents' knowledge, deal with problems, and motivate the agents. They provide the agents with a supervision schedule so that the agents will know well in advance when the supervisory visit will occur.

It can be very useful to **SET INDIVIDUAL TARGETS** for CBD agents, as they can motivate the agents and serve as a standard for evaluation. However, setting the targets must be done carefully, taking into account the following considerations:

- agents should not emphasize one contraceptive method over another just because they have a target to meet;

- targets should be tailored to the area in which the agent works, as religion, ethnicity, age, education, etc. can all affect how many people will accept family planning;

- past experience of other programs, when possible;

- the opinions and ideas of the agents themselves;

- targets should be set to achieve the desired result, for example, the contact/new client ratio is more important than just the number of contacts, and a low dropout rate is more desirable than many new acceptors of short duration.

—————————————————————————— **Momonboro** ——

TARGETS must be carefully thought out, and should be able
to be adjusted if they are not producing the desired results. At
the beginning of the CBD program in Momonboro, the agents
seemed to have attached more importance to the number of
contacts they made than to the number of acceptors they
recruited, and the supervisors let them know that the number
of acceptors was the more important of the two. In the early
stages of any such program, it will probably take a while before
the targets are adjusted to achieve exactly the right result,
taking into account the different characteristics of each agent's
district, etc.

V. COMPENSATION AND PRICING

DONE

Set PRICES

☐

Decide on method of AGENT COMPENSATION:
SALARY, COMMISSION or
COMBINATION of the two

☐

Develop BONUS SYSTEM (optional)

☐

Contraceptives should be **PRICED** (page 77) low enough to be afford-able to the poor, but probably should not be free of charge as free products are often perceived as being inferior. Even the most reason-able price will still exclude some people, and the CBD program's managers must establish a system for dealing with people who would like to use contraceptives but cannot afford them.

Momonboro

PRICING

Type of Contraceptive	CBD Price	Pharmacy Price
1 cycle of pills	M̶ 1.00	M̶ 4.50
IUD	M̶ 2.00	(not available)
Foam	M̶ .50	M̶ 19.00 per can
Condoms	Free	M̶ 1.00 for six

The pricing of contraceptives is often closely linked to the **COMPENSATION** provided to the CBD agents. In most CBD programs the agents are paid, at least in part, by receiving a percentage of the revenue they bring in. If the price is set too low, the agents will not be adequately compensated for their work and their motivation may decline.

There are several systems you can use. The advantages of providing a **FIXED SALARY** are:

- it offers the agents income security;
- it compensates all distributors equally;
- it makes it easier to attract applicants.

The disadvantages are:

- it provides little material incentive for the agents to do their work effectively;
- it gives the program little control over the quality of the distributor's work or performance.

A **STRAIGHT COMMISSION** means a distributor is paid only on the basis of his or her sales.

The advantages of this system are:

- it provides an incentive for productivity;
- it produces financial data which are directly correlated with program success.

The disadvantages of this system are:

- it does not provide an incentive for quality work;
- it does not give the agent a secure and regular income;
- it is likely to preclude the employment of full-time distributors;
- there is no guarantee that even if a distributor works hard he or she will derive any income from the work.

A **COMBINATION OF SALARY AND COMMISSION** means that the agent gets a certain amount of guaranteed money and a percentage of sales on top of that.

The advantages of this system are:

- it offers the agents income security;
- the salary makes it easier to attract applicants;
- it provides an incentive for productivity;
- it provides financial data correlated to the program's productivity.

A variation on this system is to give the agents a higher salary when the project begins and they are making their initial client contacts and have few acceptors to serve. After several months (this period of time being set in advance), when they have built up a steady and expanding clientele, the agents' salary is reduced to the regular base rate, and they have more of an incentive to recruit new acceptors.

Some programs use **BONUS** systems of awards and prizes for individual agents or teams. In judging who receives the awards, qualitative measures such as interaction with clients, community involvement, effort and cooperation can be taken into account.

Momonboro

As COMPENSATION, the CBD agents are given a salary of M20 per month, plus a 50 percent commission on all the contraceptives they sell. The team leaders, because of their greater responsibility, receive a base salary of M40 per month, and have the same arrangement on commissions.

Mrs. Tyler has also instituted an annual BONUS program, to award money to the most effective CBD agents. One prize is for the best CBD team, and is awarded on the basis of the following criteria (to be judged during monthly supervisory visits): working relationship as a group, working relationship with the community; working relationship with clients (to be judged from monthly statistics); amount of sales; and number of acceptors. The second prize goes to the six best agents, whose performance will be assessed during independent site visits by the senior management team and the executive director, who will talk with community leaders, agents and clients.

Your program must also develop procedures for dealing with indigent clients who sometimes or never can pay for their contraceptive supplies.

VI. FINANCIAL CONTROL

DONE

Develop ACCOUNTING PROCEDURES

Describe how FINANCIAL TRANSACTIONS are recorded

Create BUDGET CATEGORIES and LINE ITEMS

Project and Monitor REVENUES and EXPENSES

Develop FINANCIAL MANAGEMENT REPORTS

Every program needs an accounting system to account for money received and spent. This system must be meticulously documented, so you will need to **DEVELOP ACCOUNTING PROCEDURES** for handling and recording all financial transactions.

You must clearly **DESCRIBE HOW ALL FINANCIAL TRANSACTIONS ARE RECORDED** (page 86). The forms and instructions which will be used by the individuals who perform financial transactions must be clearly developed and documented in a financial procedures manual.

Momonboro

Mr. Armstrong set up a system which records all financial transactions of the CBD program, from the sale of contraceptives by a CBD agent to the deposit of these funds in the bank.

Projecting and monitoring expenses is an activity which is shared by the financial and program managers. They should work together to create a set of **BUDGET CATEGORIES AND LINE ITEMS** (page 87) that are flexible enough to permit **PROJECTION AND MONITORING** of all program revenues and expenses.

── **Momonboro** ──

The Chart of Accounts for the CBD project includes such budget categories as Assets, Receivables, Inventory, Fixed Assets, and Liabilities. The budget category Fixed Assets includes such line items as Office Equipment, Furniture and Fixture -- Cabinets, and Clinic Equipment -- Blood Pressure Apparatus. Mr. Armstrong uses his Expenditures Control Analysis to project and monitor the program's expenses.

Once the financial management system is operating effectively, develop **FINANCIAL MANAGEMENT REPORTS** such as in Exhibit 4 in Part VI: Financial Control. There are endless ways to use financial information to improve program management and effectiveness.

── **Momonboro** ──

The sales reports which Mr. Armstrong has developed permit him to compare program effectiveness in the different communities served by the CBD program by looking at the volume of contraceptive sales.

Summary Checklist

This checklist accompanies the Start-Up Kit. As you proceed with the kit, planning your community-based distribution program, check off on this page the tasks you have accomplished. You will be able to see at a glance how far you have advanced in setting up your program, and will be sure not to forget an essential task.

I. PLANNING

STRATEGIC PLANNING   **DONE**

    MISSION of the organization

    GOALS of the organization

    WHERE, WHAT and HOW of the organization

OPERATIONAL PLANNING

    STRATEGIES, OBJECTIVES, and TARGETS for all goals

ENVIRONMENTAL ANALYSIS

Identify:

    INTERNAL FACTORS affecting the new program

    EXTERNAL FACTORS affecting the new program

    OBSTACLES (Internal and External)

    OPPORTUNITIES (Internal and External)

Divide Obstacles into:
    Those which can be OVERCOME
    Those which can be REDUCED
    Those we must work AROUND

Identify PROBLEMS which could occur and PROPOSED SOLUTIONS

DONE

Develop a LIST OF PEOPLE WHO CAN INFLUENCE THE PROGRAM'S SUCCESS

Meet with the people on this LIST

Get the support of COMMUNITY LEADERS

II. DEVELOPING THE PROGRAM

Involve your STAFF

Conduct NEEDS ASSESSMENT of the community

Select CBD AGENTS

Train CBD AGENTS

Set up RESUPPLY SYSTEM

Choose CONTRACEPTIVE METHODS to distribute

III.   MANAGEMENT INFORMATION SYSTEM

Identify INFORMATION USERS at every level

Identify INFORMATION needed at every level

Identify HOW MANAGERS WILL USE THE INFORMATION
     Evaluation of CBD agents and of the program
     Indicators of program performance

Design DATA COLLECTION FORMS

Design REPORTING FORMATS for all levels

Train AGENTS, TEAM LEADERS AND SUPERVISORS
to collect, report and analyze information at their level

DONE

IV. SUPERVISION

Build a SUPERVISORY STRUCTURE

Develop a SUPERVISORY SCHEDULE

Provide REGULAR FEEDBACK

Set TARGETS for CBD agents

V. COMPENSATION AND PRICING

Set PRICES

Decide on method of AGENT COMPENSATION: SALARY, COMMISSION, or COMBINATION of the two

Develop BONUS SYSTEM (optional)

VI. FINANCIAL CONTROL

Develop ACCOUNTING PROCEDURES

Describe how FINANCIAL TRANSACTIONS are recorded

Create BUDGET CATEGORIES and LINE ITEMS

Project and Monitor REVENUES and EXPENSES

Develop FINANCIAL MANAGEMENT REPORTS

ANNEX 1

Chronology of Events: The Community-Based Distribution Process in Momonboro

<u>Years One and Two</u>

Mrs. Tyler becomes Executive Director of the Family Planning Association of Momonboro.

FPAM undergoes organizational restructuring. The Board of FPAM broadens the role of the statistical officer to include program evaluation. Mr. William Alphonse is hired for this new position.

Mrs. Tyler visits communities to judge the level of contraceptive awareness.

<u>Year Three</u>

Team of consultants comes to review the country's experiences in population and family planning. They recommend a community-based distribution program.

Mr. Ford and Mrs. Tyler decide that an outreach and community-based distribution program would help FPAM reach more families.

Mrs. Tyler writes to international family planning funding agencies about her proposed CBD program.

Professor Pedipaw of Pathways meets with FPAM, reviews the current situation and drafts guidelines for a proposal. He requests that FPAM conduct a needs assessment in the planned project service area.

Mrs. Tyler and the staff select six potential communities for the CBD program, and send out a survey questionnaire to the mayor of each community.

FPAM holds a meeting of the mayors and commissioners of each community to discuss the survey results, to outline the plans for the CBD project, and to ask for the suggestions and help of the mayors and commissioners.

FPAM holds meetings with officials from the Ministry of Health and eliminate barriers to the program.

Mr. Alphonse develops a management information system for the CBD program.

Year Four

Two Pathways representatives arrive to help FPAM develop the final draft of the proposal. The consultants visit the Ministries which are connected with the project.

The CBD project receives final approval for funding.

Year Five

The new financial officer, Mr. Louis Armstrong, begins his work at FPAM and sets up a financial control system for the CBD project.

Detailed plans for the MIS are begun in a training workshop. Participants design the CBD agent record, team leader's monthly report form, and the CBD officer's monthly report form.

The CBD agents are trained.

The CBD agents begin working in their communities.

ANNEX 2

Sample Job Descriptions

Community-Based Distribution Project Officer

Job Title	CBD Project Officer
Department	Community-Based Distribution Project
Reports to	Project Director

Job Summary
Supervise all aspects of the CBD program (performance of agents and meeting of targets) and maintain close relations with the communities and other parties involved.

Job Responsibilities
Maintain good working relations with the community, government agencies, individuals and institutions involved in family planning work in Momonboro.

Review program operations regularly and identify and correct performance problems.

Review all monthly reports including financial computations.

Hold joint monthly meetings with CBD workers and team leaders and review the progress of the work; check records and carry out spot verification of distributors' and team leaders' monthly performance.

Impart routine training to distributors during supervisory meetings and monitor project's progress.

Provide feedback on distributors' performance to area community leaders and obtain periodic information on community's response to the program.

Coordinate the activities and input of all the other units of the FPAM and from consultants.

Qualifications
Minimum first degree in social science or nursing with experience in social work, family planning, or community development.
Area resident but with ability to travel independently.
Ability to communicate well in English and one of the local languages.
Minimum of thirty years of age.

Attitudes and Personal Qualities
Female, preferably married.
Good personality.

Community-Based Distribution Project Junior Accountant

Job title   CBD Junior Accountant
Department   CBD Project
Reports to   Finance Officer

Job Summary
Work with the finance staff in setting up and maintaining the books of accounts on the project and prepare financial summaries and monthly reports.

Job Responsibilities
Prepare payment vouchers.

Write up cash payment and cash receipt books.

Write up petty cash book.

Post the general ledger and take up trial balances monthly.

Reconcile the monthly bank statements.

Maintain a daily cash book.

Maintain vendors and debtors subsidiary ledgers.

Perform other duties that may be determined from time to time by the superior officers.

Is subject at all times to the directive of the Executive Director of FPAM who is the Project Director.

Qualifications
High school graduate or above.
Diploma in accounting or its equivalent.
Two years practical experience in accounting work.
A college education will be an advantage.
Ability to work independently.
Ability to analyze, synthesize, perceive, and report with clarity.

Attitudes and Personal Qualities
Ability to work under pressure and for long hours.

Community-Based Distribution Assistant Evaluation Officer

Job title   CBD Assistant Evaluation Officer
Department   Community-Based Distribution Project
Reports to   Evaluation Officer

Job Summary
Perform evaluation and other tasks for the CBD Project to support the work of the Evaluation Officer.

Job Responsibilities
Receive, tabulate, and analyze the field returns from the CBD Project under the supervision of the Evaluation Officer.

Assist the Evaluation Officer in formulating the overall plan for the Unit.

Assist other personnel in the development of a realistic and measurable work program budget, three year plan, and other action strategies.

Serve as the principal deputy to the Evaluation Officer and will advise her or him on matters relating to the CBD project.

Undertake any other task that may be given to her or him by the Project Director.

Qualifications
A university degree in demography, education, economics, statistics, or advanced studies.
Experience and capability in research and evaluation.
Two years of work experience.
Ability to develop research proposals and evaluation guidelines.
Ability to speak and write English fluently.

Attitudes and Personal Qualities
Ability to work under pressure and for long hours.

Community-Based Distribution Project Secretary

Job Title   CBD Secretary
Department   CBD Project
Reports to   National Program Coordinator

Job Summary
Generally responsible for typing all communications regarding the CBD project activities implementation: taking minutes at meetings with agents, program committee members and FPAM executive meetings, community centers/information out going from CBD/FPAM staff relating to CBD, and other assigned tasks as relates to a Secretary in the office.

Job Responsibilities
Responsible to Project Coordinator/FPAM Administrative/Personnel Officer

Serve as secretary to the Project Director and Accountant.

Type all communications relating to CBD activities.

Type monthly and quarterly progress reports of CBD activities and dispatch them to divisional head for signature.

Keep confidential and other files placed in secretary's possession up to date.

Receive and dispatch important and all FPAM/CBD mail in secretary's care.

Maintain the attendance of the project staff.

Operate FPAM photocopy and mimeograph machines.

Take minutes at all meetings, type them, and distribute them to office personnel and CBD agents and program committee members and other community leaders.

Do all other assignments delegated to the secretary by the Project Director, the National Program Coordinator.

Demonstrate interest in the activity and performance of the FPAM and the CBD project.

Qualifications
High school graduate and must have completed a recognized secretarial institution. Two years of working experience.

Attitudes and Personal Qualities
Must be pleasant, well groomed, trustworthy, honest.
A Momonborian

Driver for Community-Based Distribution Project

Job title   Driver for CBD project
Department   CBD project
Reports to   FPAM Administrative and Personnel Officer

Job Summary
Responsible for transporting staff, agents, and program committee members as necessary and for the operation and upkeep of vehicles and other equipment.

Job Responsibilities
Transport staff to project areas. Transport agents and program committee members to supervisory and monitoring visits.

Take agents to practical areas during field trip.

Dispatch and deliver mail upon directives from Project Director, Coordinator, Program Officers, Secretary.

Keep assigned vehicle clean, keep daily log book of vehicles up to date, and report all mechanical problems immediately for necessary repairs.

Learn to operate projector and the program machines.

Carry supplies/equipment to and from vehicle when need arises.

Demonstrate interest in the advancement of FPAM and the CBD project.

Perform other duties as may be assigned by the Administrative and Personnel Officer.

Qualifications
At least junior high school.
Two years of driving experience with some knowledge of vehicle maintenance.
Momonborian with valid Momonborian driving license.
Ability to take and follow instructions.
Able to work long hours.

Attitudes and Personal Qualities
Honest, obedient and trustworthy.
Pleasant and neat appearance.

Community-Based Distribution Team Leader

Job Title   CBD Team Leader
Department   CBD Project
Reports to   Program Committee Member/CBD Project Officer

Job Summary
Supervise CBD agents and report to CBD Program Officer

Job Responsibilities
Coordinate, supervise, and monitor the CBD agents in Team Leader's specified area.

Responsible to the CBD Program Officer for all nonfinancial matters. Responsible to the Junior Accountant for all financial matters.

Map out the area of responsibility of each CBD agent and ensure it is adhered to.

Assist distributors in setting targets for IEC acceptors and referrals.

Maintain accurate and up-to-date accounts of the sales of contraceptives.

Check up on effectiveness of referrals of clients to clinic at CBD agents' level.

Qualifications
At least 7th grade.
Must be a CBD agent and therefore fulfill those conditions and job descriptions.

Community-Based Distribution Agent

Job Title   CBD Agent
Department   CBD Project
Reports to   CBD Team Leader

Job Summary
To promote information, education and communication of family planning within the communities to individual couples and groups of the community. To recruit and serve family planning acceptors.

Job Responsibilities
Make at least sixty contacts per month.

Distribute pills, foaming tablets and condoms to eligible clients. Store all contraceptives safely. Recruit at least six new acceptors per month.

Refer clients to approved backup clinics for oral contraceptives and injectables. Make at least six referrals a month.

Report all funds for sales to Team Leader, of which 50 percent will be returned and the necessary receipt obtained. Responsible to the Team Leader for program and finances.

Prepare all required reports and keep records.

Follow-up on clients, both referred to clinic and non-referral, at community level.

Work with other CBD agents in the team to avoid duplication of clients and overlapping of work zones.

Responsible to the Purchase and Supply Officer.

Comply with the schedule of reports and supervisory visits.

Qualifications
At least 7th grade.
Ability to speak at least one local language of assigned community.
Must be nominated by the Local Project Area Committee.
Demonstrated interest in Family Planning by previous or present practicing of a method.

Attitudes and Personal Qualities
Mature and respected member of the community.

ANNEX 3

Sample Forms

FPAM/CBD Agent's Client Record Form

Name of Client: _____
Address: _____ Zone: _____
_____

Background Information

Age: _____ Number of living children: _____

Sex: _____ Ever use contraceptive? (Yes/No)

Ed. attained: _____ If yes, method: _____

Year	JAN	FEB	MAR	APR	MAY	JUN	JUL	AUG	SEP	OCT	NOV	DEC
19												
19												
19												
19												
19												

Codes

Methods given	Referrals made	Dropout reasons
LF=LoFemenal	R1=Pill	D1=Wants child
OV=Ovral	R2=IUD	D2=Pregnant
MY=Mycrogynon	R3=Depo provera	D3=Side effects
N=Nordette	R4=Sterilization	D4=Husband against
MA=Marvelon	R5=Medical exam	D5=Medical reasons
FT=Foam tablet	R6=Side effects	D6=Migration
C=Condom	R7=Infertility	D7=Others
FC=Foam cream	R8=Others	

FPAM/CBD
Client Referral Card

Part I   Serial No. _____

Client Name: _____

Zone: _____

Type of service desired:
(circle all that apply)

1. Contraceptive
2. Lab test
3. Medical exam
4. Post partum
5. Nutrition
6. Gynecological
7. Infertility
8. Sterilization: ☐ M ☐ F

Referral Date: _____

Agent's Name: _____

Area: _____

This side should be filled out and kept by the CBD Agent.

FPAM/CBD
Client Referral Card

Part II   Serial No. _____

Dear Nurse Midwife: _____

I have referred _____
                          (client's name)

to you for:

1. Contraceptive   5. Nutrition
2. Lab test   6. Gynecological
3. Medical exam   7. Infertility
4. Post partum   8. Sterilization
                         ☐ M ☐ F

Agent's Name: _____

To be completed by FPAM Nurse:

Date of visit: _____

Type of service provided:

1. Contraceptive   5. Nutrition
2. Lab test   6. Gynecological
3. Medical exam   7. Infertility
4. Post partum   8. Sterilization
                         ☐ M ☐ F

Family planning method given: _____

Family planning visit card no.: _____

I certify that this client received the service above.

Signed: _____

Date: _____   Clinic/area: _____

This side should be given to the client to take to the clinic

FPAM/CBD Agent's Monthly Worksheet
(To be completed with Team Leader)

Agent Name: _____   Area: _____   Month: _____

Date: _____   Year: _____

I Number of New Users (one tick for each new user)									Total
Pills	ooooo	ooooo	ooooo	ooooo	ooooo	ooooo	ooooo	ooooo	
Condoms	ooooo	ooooo	ooooo	ooooo	ooooo	ooooo	ooooo	ooooo	
Foam can	ooooo	ooooo	ooooo	ooooo	ooooo	ooooo	ooooo	ooooo	
Foam tablet	ooooo	ooooo	ooooo	ooooo	ooooo	ooooo	ooooo	ooooo	

II Contraceptives Distributed (one tick for each cycle or can; write in number of units for condoms and foam tablets)									Total
Pills	ooooo	ooooo	ooooo	ooooo	ooooo	ooooo	ooooo	ooooo	
Condoms									
Foam tablets									
Foam cream	ooooo	ooooo	ooooo	ooooo	ooooo	ooooo	ooooo	ooooo	

III Referral Made (one tick for each referral made)									Total
Pills	ooooo	ooooo	ooooo	ooooo	ooooo	ooooo	ooooo	ooooo	
IUD	ooooo	ooooo	ooooo	ooooo	ooooo	ooooo	ooooo	ooooo	
Injectable	ooooo	ooooo	ooooo	ooooo	ooooo	ooooo	ooooo	ooooo	
Sterilization (M)	ooooo	ooooo	ooooo	ooooo	ooooo	ooooo	ooooo	ooooo	
Sterilization (F)	ooooo	ooooo	ooooo	ooooo	ooooo	ooooo	ooooo	ooooo	
Other	ooooo	ooooo	ooooo	ooooo	ooooo	ooooo	ooooo	ooooo	

IV Dropouts (one tick for each dropout)									Total
Side effects	ooooo	ooooo	ooooo	ooooo	ooooo	ooooo	ooooo	ooooo	
Pregnancy	ooooo	ooooo	ooooo	ooooo	ooooo	ooooo	ooooo	ooooo	
Medical	ooooo	ooooo	ooooo	ooooo	ooooo	ooooo	ooooo	ooooo	
Other	ooooo	ooooo	ooooo	ooooo	ooooo	ooooo	ooooo	ooooo	

FPAM/CBD Agent's Monthly Totals
(To be completed by Team Leader)

Agent's Name: _____   Area: _____   Year: ____

I	No. of new users	JAN	FEB	MAR	APR	MAY	JUN	JUL	AUG	SEP	OCT	NOV	DEC
	Pills												
	Condom												
	Foam tablet												
	Foam can												

II	Contraceptives distributed												
	Pills												
	Condom												
	Foam tablet												
	Foam can												

III	Number of referrals												
	Pills												
	IUD												
	Injectable												
	Sterilization (M)												
	Sterilization (F)												
	Medical exam												
	Other												

IV	Number of dropouts												
	Side effects												
	Pregnancy												
	Medical												
	Other												

Team Leader's name: _____

ANNEX 4

Training Program for Community-Based Distribution Agents

The Family Planning Association of Momonboro has conducted a number of training activities intended to improve the awareness of the project staff and the CBD agents about family planning issues. Much of the training which the FPAM has done involves preparing CBD agents for their role in the project. Among these activities have been:

- A community-based distribution observation tour. The FPAM Legal Advisor, Program Officers for Service Delivery and Information, Education and Communication (IEC), and the CBD Project Coordinator went on this tour to become familiar with the operation of a CBD project.

- Training of community leaders and program committee members.

- Training of community-based distribution trainers.

- Training of CBD volunteers.

- Refresher training of CBD volunteers.

- Training the CBD Secretary and two other FPAM staff members in the use of the microcomputers.

- Update training for Referral Backup Clinic Staff.

- Training of new CBD agents.

- Training of twenty CBD agents and six CBD/FPAM staff on the development of IEC materials for readers and non-readers.

Training of CBD Agents

The new CBD agents are trained by a team of FPAM staff, consisting of the National Program Coordinator, the CBD Program Officer, the Program Officer for Service Delivery, the IEC Officer, and the Evaluation Officer. Often, this team is complemented by resource people from Momonboro's Ministry of Health. The training course is two weeks long.

The training curriculum for new CBD agents includes the following topics:

- The Aims and Objectives of the CBD Project;
- The Benefits of Family Planning;
- Basic Human Reproduction;
- Family Planning Methods;
- Side Effects, Contraindications, and Complications;
- Family Planning Information and Education;
- Screening and Counseling of Potential Clients;
- Follow-up Visits and Client Referrals;
- Distribution of Contraceptives Using a Checklist;
- Responsibilities of CBD workers;
- Community and Household Mapping;
- Dealing with Rumors in Family Planning.

The training program emphasizes practical skills, and trainers use group discussions, role-play activities, and pictorial presentations to relay the information. The training team then assesses how well the agents have learned the skills and tests them on how well they counsel clients, communicate family planning information to clients, use the oral contraceptive checklist, and conduct follow-up procedures and bookkeeping. The trainers assess these skills through role playing exercises and field practice. The agents who have sufficiently learned these skills receive a certificate in a ceremony which is conducted in their area. The training program is evaluated through the use of questionnaires, observation, and personal interviews.

The CBD team leaders receive an additional two to three days of training on community mapping, target setting, supervision, reporting and basic accounting.

After several months, the CBD agents and team leaders are given refresher training. In group discussions, they share their experiences and identify and discuss common problems and ways to deal with them. These discussions also help the trainers to identify any existing deficiencies in the training curriculum or in the training methods used.

Refresher sessions and more recent training sessions have included discussions on the following additional topics:

- Sexually transmitted diseases, including AIDS;
- Information and education on high risk young adults;
- Oral rehydration therapy;
- Immunization;
- Breast feeding;
- Record-keeping with emphasis on newly developed recording/reporting forms.

ANNEX 5

Flipchart for Family Planning Presentation

This flipchart was developed by the Family Planning Association of Momonboro for use by the CBD agents on their home visits.

Content of Flipchart

1. General Family Planning Information

   - Definition

   - Benefits (health, education, financial, time)

   - Traditional versus Modern Methods

2. Counseling

   - Tell clients about their individual rights to family planning services:

     - Clients have a right to choose the method best for them
     - Clients have the right to change their method if necessary

   - Tell clients about individual differences in body makeup

   - Each couple may choose a different contraceptive method

3. Female Reproductive Organs
   Tell clients that the picture is of the part of the woman's body which is responsible for childbearing

   - Name the various parts, that is, vagina, cervix, womb, Fallopian tubes, ovaries

   - Tell the functions of each part (short notes)

   - Explain the process of the ovary storing eggs, releasing eggs monthly, fertilization, pregnancy, if conception doesn't occur menstruation takes place and the uterus forms a new lining

4. Male Reproductive Organs
   (Procedure as for female organs)

5. Contraceptive Methods Available from CBD project (three main methods)

- Pill
- Condom
- Foam Cream/Tablet

Information on *How They Work, Advantages and Disadvantages*

6. Other Clinical Methods

- IUD
- Injectable
- Vasectomy
- Tubal Ligation

Information on *How They Work, Advantages and Disadvantages*

ANNEX 6

CBD Agent's Oral Contraceptive Checklist

This checklist was developed by the Family Planning Association of Momonboro to help the CBD agents identify suitable candidates for the oral contraceptive pill.

Objectives

1. To enable CBD agents to select the suitable child spacing and family planning method for the client.

2. To identify clients for referral to a health center.

When to Use the Pill Checklist

The CBD agent uses the checklist when:

- a client has decided to use a method of child spacing/family planning;

- switching a breastfeeding client from Progestin-Only Pills to Combined Oral Contraceptives;

- restarting a client who has stopped using family planning;

- resupplying a client who has no child spacing/family planning card to show what pill she has been taking.

How to Use the Pill Checklist

The CBD agent must cover all the items on the checklist, starting at the beginning and going in order to the end, recording any positive responses on the right.

	YES
Do not give either Combined Oral Contraceptives or Progestin Only Pills if the answer is "YES" to **any** of the following questions:	
1a. Did you miss your last period? (Ask only if the woman is not breastfeeding.) If the answer is yes, ask her question b. If the answer is no, proceed to question 2.	☐
b. After missing your period, have you had any unusual bleeding?	☐
2. How old are you?	
3. Do you bleed after sexual intercourse?	☐
4. Do you have any unusual bleeding between your periods?	☐
5. Have you ever experienced a severe sharp pain at the back of either of your legs?	☐
6. Have you ever experienced a severe sharp pain in your chest that made it difficult for you to breathe?	☐
7. Have your eyes and palms turned yellow in the past twelve months?	☐
8. Have you experienced shortness of breath after walking a short distance or doing some light work?	☐
9. Have you had severe headaches that do not get better after taking Cafenol or Aspirin?	☐

If the answer is yes to any of these questions (except question 2), the client needs to be checked at a health center. Therefore you should give her a referral slip and refer her to the health center. Give her condoms for her husband in the meantime.

BIBLIOGRAPHY

Anthony, Robert, and David Young. *Management Control in Non-Profit Organizations*. Homewood, IL: Irwin, 1984.

Beeson, Diane, M. Faith Mitchell, Helene Lipton, Donald Minkler, Philip R. Lee. "Client Provider Transactions in Community-Based Family Planning Programs and the Outreach Component of Clinic-Based Programs," in *Organizing for Effective Family Planning Programs*, Robert J. Lapham and George B. Simmonds, Editors. Washington, DC: National Academy Press, 1987.

Cuca, Roberto, and Catherine S. Pierce. *Experiments in Family Planning*. Baltimore: Johns Hopkins University Press, 1977.

David, Henry P. "Incentives and Disincentives in Family Planning Programs," in Lapham and Simmons, eds., pp. 521-542.

David, Henry P. *Incentives, Fertility Behavior, and Integrated Community Development: An Overview*. Bethesda: Transnational Family Research Institute, 1980, monograph.

Foreit, J.R., and K. Foreit. "Quarterly versus Monthly Supervision of CBD Family Planning Programs: An Experimental Study in Northeast Brazil," *Studies in Family Planning*, 15(3):112-120.

Foreit, J.R., et al. "Community-Based and Commercial Contraceptive Distribution: An Inventory and Appraisal," *Population Reports*, Series J, No. 19. Baltimore, MD: The Johns Hopkins University Press, 1978.

Gray, R.H., and M.H. Labbock. "Family Planning Components in Community-Based Distribution Projects: Risk/Benefit Consideration and in the Choice of Methods," in *Health and Family Planning in Community-Based Distribution Programs*, Maria Wawer, Sandra Huffman, Deborah Cebula and Richard Osborn, eds., pp. 65-104. Boulder, CO: Westview Press, 1985.

Hatcher, Robert A., et al, *Family Planning Methods and Practice: Africa*. Richardson, TX: Christian Medical Society, 1984.

Herm, James. "Worker and Manager Accountability," in Lapham and Simmons, eds., 263-294.

Huber, S.C., et al. "Contraceptive Distribution: Taking Supplies to Villages and Households," *Population Reports*, Series J, No. 5. Baltimore, MD: The Johns Hopkins University Press, 1975.

Jain, Sagar C., K. Kanagaratnam, and John Paul, Eds. *Management Development in Population Programs*. Chapel Hill, NC: University of North Carolina and Carolina Population Center, 1981.

Kols, A.J., and M.J. Wawer. "Community-Based Health and Family Planning," *Population Reports*, Series L-3, No. 10(6). Baltimore, MD: The Johns Hopkins University Press, 1982.

Korten, David C. "Management Issues in the Organization and Delivery of Family Planning Services: International Perspective." Paper presented at the 104th Annual Meeting of the American Public Health Association, October 17-21, 1976, Miami Beach, Florida.

Korten, David C. "Managing Community-Based Population Programmes: Insights from the 1978 ICOMP Annual Conference." Kuala Lumpur, Malaysia, July 17-19, 1978.

Korten, Francis F. and David C. Korten. *Casebook for Family Planning Management*. Boston, MA: The Pathfinder Fund, 1977.

Lapham, Robert J., and George B. Simmons, eds. *Organizing for Effective Family Planning Programs*. Washington, DC: National Academy Press, 1987.

Mayo-Smith, Ian. *Managing People: Five International Case Studies*. West Hartford, CT: Kumarian Press, 1983.

Osborn, R.W., and W.A. Reinke, eds. *Community-Based Distribution of Contraception: A Review of Field Experience*. Baltimore, MD: The Johns Hopkins University Population Center, 1981.

Rosenfield, A. "Auxiliaries and Family Planning," *Lancet* 1 (7855):443.

Ross, John A. *Family Planning Pilot Projects in Africa: Review and Synthesis*. Washington, DC: World Bank, PHN Technical Note 85-7, 1985.

Ross, John A. and Stephen L. Isaacs. "Costs, Payments, and Incentives in Family Planning Programs: A Review of Developing Countries," *Studies in Family Planning* 19:5 (1988):270-283.

Ross, John A., Donald D. Lauro, Joe D. Wray and Allan G. Rosenfield. "Community-Based Distribution," in Lapham and Simmons, eds., pp. 343-366.

Talpaert, Roger. *Managing a Management Development Institution*. Geneva: ILO, 1982.

Trainer, E.S. "Community-Based Integrated Family Planning Programs," *Studies in Family Planning* 10(5):177-182.

Vernon, Ricardo, Gabriel Ojeda and Marcia C. Townsend. "Contraceptive Social Marketing and Community-Based Distribution Systems in Colombia," *Studies in Family Planning* 19(6):354-360.

Warwick, Donald P. *Bitter Pills*. Cambridge: Cambridge University Press, 1982.

Wortman, J. "Training Non-physicians in Family Planning Services," *Population Reports*. Series J, No. 6. Baltimore, MD: The Johns Hopkins University Press, 1975.

INDEX

Accounting system, 86-87

Budget, 87

Chart of accounts, 87, 100-101

Chronology of events, 140-141

Community-Based Distribution, goal of, 1

    reasons for, 23

    socio-cultural implications of, 5

Community-Based Distribution Agent, data collection form of, 49

    information collected by, 45

    job description of, 148

    remuneration, 3, 67, 77-78, 80-81

    responsibilities of, 45

    selection, 2

    supervision of, 3, 66-68

    training, 2

Community-Based Distribution Project Assistant Evaluation Officer, job description of, 144

Community-Based Distribution Project Driver, job description of, 146

Community-Based Distribution Project Junior Accountant, job description of, 143

Community-Based Distribution Project Officer, data collection form of, 51

    information collected by, 46

    job description of, 142

    responsibilities of, 46

Community-Based Distribution Project Secretary, job description of, 145

Community-Based Distribution Start-up Kit, 106-139

Community-Based Distribution Team Leader, data collection form of, 50

    information collected by, 46

    job description of, 147

    responsibilities of, 45

Community leaders, support of, 2, 29-30, 35

Community support, 2, 29-30

Contraceptive method mix, 4

Contraceptive pricing, 4, 77

Environmental analysis, 12-13

Evaluation, 38-39, 52-53

Family Planning Association of Momonboro, 8

    organization of, 8-9

Feedback, 40, 46, 59, 66-67

Financial management, 86-88

Financial statement, 86

Flipchart for presentation, 156

Forms for data collection, 40, 49-51

Goals of an organization, 11

Indicators, 39, 46, 59

Information, Education, and Communication (IEC), 8

Management information system (MIS), design of, 37-38, 64

Ministry of Health, Momonboro, 7

Mission of an organization, 11

Mix of services, 4

Needs assessment, 2, 28-29

Objectives in operational planning, 11

Operational planning, 11

Oral contraceptive checklist, 158

Planning, 10, 35-36

Ratios, 58

Receipt of sale, 96

Resupply system, 3

Staff involvement in program design, 11

Stock control form, 97

Strategic planning, 10-11

Strategy in operational planning, 11

Survey of potential communities, 33

Supervision, 3, 66-68

Targets, 11, 39, 58-59

About the authors

James A. Wolff is currently the Director of Special Projects for the Family Planning Management Training Program at Management Sciences for Health. For the past twelve years he has been actively involved in assisting both public and private sector health and family planning organizations in countries throughout the world to improve their management. Dr. Wolff is an adjunct associate professor of Health Services at Boston University School of Medicine and has been a consultant with USAID, WHO, and the World Bank. He received a B.A. from Harvard College, a B.M.S. from Dartmouth College, an M.D. from Columbia University College of Physicians and Surgeons, and an M.A.T. and M.P.H. from Harvard University. In addition to his management work and teaching, Dr. Wolff practices emergency medicine in Boston.

Robert Cushman, Jr., is affiliated with Dalhousie Health and Community Services in Ottawa, Canada, where he conducts clinical work and epidemiology. He is involved in the provision and organization of family planning services in Ottawa. He has extensive experience in Africa, ranging from clinical work in Zambia to program planning and evaluation in Liberia and Senegal. Dr. Cushman received his B.A. from Harvard College and his M.D. and M.S. from MacMaster University. Dr. Cushman has written several papers on the effectiveness and impact of preventive strategies on health.

Florida A. Kweekeh has worked in the fields of health education and family planning information and management for almost twenty years. She is a member of the Program Review and Finance Committee of the International Family Planning Federation, Africa Region, which makes major program direction decisions for family planning associations in the Africa region. At present, she is the Executive Director of the Cuttington University College Centennial Fund Drive in Liberia. Ms. Kweekeh received a B.S. degree from Cuttington University College in Liberia, and an M.P.H. from the University of Ibadan in Nigeria. Ms. Kweekeh's expertise includes health communications, and she has written several health dramas for radio broadcast.

C. Elizabeth McGrory is currently the Assistant Director of the World Population Program at the John D. and Catherine T. MacArthur Foundation. She has worked with programs providing health care, development assistance, research and study opportunities, and family planning assistance. Ms. McGrory received an A.B. degree in International Development Studies from Brown University and an Sc.M. in Health Policy and Management from Harvard University. Ms. McGrory is particularly interested in women's health and rights in developing countries.

Susanna C. Binzen is the Special Projects Associate at Management Sciences for Health, where she is an editor and writer of a variety of materials on family planning program management, including a basic family planning management handbook. She has worked with a number of organizations to increase public awareness on the issues of world population and family planning. Ms. Binzen received a B.S.F.S. degree from Georgetown University School of Foreign Service and an M.P.H. from Columbia University. Ms. Binzen has a strong interest in world population growth and its impact on the environment, and is actively involved in local environmental efforts.